Adler • Beckers • Buck **PNF in Practice**

ERSITY OF
GHAM

Springer
Berlin
Heidelberg
New York
Hong Kong
London
Milan
Paris
Tokyo

S. S. Adler   D. Beckers
M. Buck

PNF in Practice

An Illustrated Guide

Second, revised edition

With 209 Figures in 558 Separate Illustrations

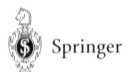 Springer

Susan S. Adler
161 E Chicago Ave, Apt 35E
Chicago, IL 60611
USA

Dominiek Beckers
Rehabilitation Centre Hoensbroek
Zandbergsweg 111
NL-6432 CC Hoensbroek

Math Buck
Rehabilitation Centre Hoensbroek
Zandbergsweg 111
NL-6432 CC Hoensbroek

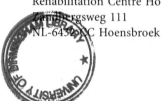

2nd corr. printing 2003

ISBN 3-540-66395-9 Springer-Verlag Berlin Heidelberg New York

Library of Congress Cataloging-in-Publication Data
Die Deutsche Bibliothek – CIP-Einheitsaufnahme
Adler, Susan S.: PNF in practice: an illustrated guide/Susan S. Adler; Dominiek Beckers;
Math Buck. – 2. ed. – Berlin; Heidelberg; New York; Barcelona; Hong Kong; London;
Milan; Paris; Singapore; Tokyo: Springer, 1999
     ISBN 3-540-66395-9

Production: PRO EDIT GmbH, 69126 Heidelberg, Germany
Typesetting (Data conversion): K+V Fotosatz GmbH, 64743 Beerfelden, Germany
Cover Design: Künkel + Lopka Werbeagentur, 69123 Heidelberg, Germany

Printed on acid-free paper   SPIN 11402244   22/3111/is – 5 4 3 2

To Maggie Knott, teacher and friend.

Devoted to her patients,
dedicated to her students,
a pioneer in profession

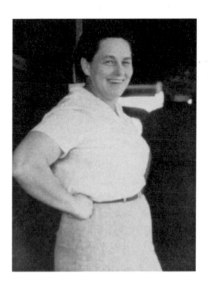

Preface

Proprioceptive neuromuscular facilitation (PNF) is a philosophy and a method of treatment. It was started by *Dr. Herman Kabat* in the 1940s. Dr. Kabat and *Margaret (Maggie) Knott* continued to expand and develop the treatment techniques and procedures after their move to Vallejo, California in 1947. After *Dorothy Voss* joined the team in 1953, Maggie and Dorothy wrote the first PNF book, published in 1956. Dr. Sedgewick Mead, who replaced Dr. Kabat, supported the continued growth of the PNF concept. At first PNF was used as treatment for patients with poliomyelitis. With experience it became clear that this treatment approach was effective for patients with a wide range of diagnoses.

The three- and six-month PNF courses in Vallejo began in the 1950s. Physical therapists from all over the world have journeyed to Vallejo to learn the theoretical and practical aspects of the PNF concept. In addition, Knott and Voss traveled in the United States and abroad to give introductory courses in the concept.

When Maggie Knott died in 1978 her work at Vallejo was carried on by Carolyn Oei Hvistendahl, who is now living in Norway. Carolyn was succeeded by Hink Mangold as director of the PNF program until her retirement in 1998. Tim Josten is the present program director. Sue Adler, Gregg Johnson, and Vicky Saliba have also continued Maggie's work as teachers of the PNF concept. Sue Adler designed the Advanced and Instructor course programs of the International PNF Association (IPNFA).

Developments in the PNF concept are closely followed throughout the world. It is now possible to take recognized training courses in many countries given by qualified PNF instructors.

The material in this book is based on treatment innovations begun by Dr. Herman Kabat and expanded by Margaret Knott, Dorothy Voss, and others, both therapists and patients. The authors acknowledge their debt to these outstanding people, and also to all members of the IPNFA, and hope that this book will encourage others to carry on the work.

There are other excellent books dealing with the PNF method, but they are all general works providing an extensive theoretical description of the treatment. We felt there was a need for a comprehensive coverage of the practical techniques in text and illustrations. This book should thus be seen as a practical guide and used in combination with existing textbooks. We recommend further reading in both the second and third editions of the book "Proprioceptive Neuromuscular Facilitation: Patterns and Techniques" by Knott and Voss (1968), and Voss, Ionta and Meyers (1985), respectively, as well as the works by Sullivan et al. (1982), Sullivan and Marcos (1995), and by Hedin-Andén (1994).

This book would not have been possible without the cooperation of the Stichting voor Revalidatie Limburg in Hoensbroek (The Netherlands). A special note of thanks goes to the following: F. Somers for the photography, colleague José van Oppen for acting as a model, Jan Albers for assistance in organization and Ben Eisermann for the drawings. We also wish to thank Christina Kessler and Morgan Rose for acting as models for the scapula and pelvis pictures, and Erwin Punz for the photography.

And, finally, we are grateful to all our patients. A special word of appreciation is owed the patients acting as model in this new edition.

Autumn 1999   S. S. Adler, D. Beckers, M. Buck

References

Hedin-Andén S (1994) PNF-Grundverfahren und Funktionelles Training. Bank und Mattentraining, Gangschulung. Gustav Fischer, Stuttgart

Knott M, Voss DE (1968) Proprioceptive Neuromuscular Facilitation, patterns and techniques, 2nd edn. Harper and Row, New York

Sullivan PE, Markos PD (1995) Clinical decision making in therapeutic exercise. Appleton and Lange, Norwalk, CT

Sullivan PE, Markos PD, Minor MAD (1982) An integrated approach to therapeutic exercise, theory and clinical application. Reston Publishing Company, Reston, Va

Voss DE, Ionta M, Meyers B (1985) Proprioceptive Neuromuscular Facilitation, patterns and techniques, 3rd edn. Harper and Row, New York

Contents

1	**Introduction to Proprioceptive Neuromuscular Facilitation**	1

2	**Basic Procedures for Facilitation**	3
2.1	Resistance	4
2.2	Irradiation and Reinforcement	6
2.3	Manual Contact	8
2.4	Body Position and Body Mechanics	10
2.5	Verbal Stimulation (Commands)	10
2.6	Vision	11
2.7	Traction and Approximation	12
2.8	Stretch	13
2.9	Timing	15
2.10	Patterns	17

3	**Techniques**	19
3.1	Rhythmic Initiation	20
3.2	Combination of Isotonics	22
3.3	Reversal of Antagonists	24
3.3.1	Dynamic Reversals	24
3.3.2	Stabilizing Reversals	28
3.3.3	Rhythmic Stabilization	31
3.4	Repeated Stretch (Repeated Contractions)	33
3.4.1	Repeated Stretch from Beginning of Range	33
3.4.2	Repeated Stretch Through Range	35
3.5	Contract-Relax	38
3.5.1	Contract-Relax: Direct Treatment	38
3.5.2	Contract-Relax: Indirect Treatment	40
3.6	Hold-Relax	40
3.6.1	Hold-Relax: Direct Treatment	40
3.6.2	Hold-Relax: Indirect Treatment	42
3.7	Replication	43
3.8	PNF Techniques and Their Goals	44

4   Patient Treatment 47
4.1   Evaluation 47
4.2   Treatment Goals 48
4.3   Treatment Planning and Treatment Design 49
4.3.1   Specific Patient Needs 49
4.3.2   Designing the Treatment 49
4.4   Assessment 50
4.5   Direct and Indirect Treatment 50
4.5.1   Direct Treatment 50
4.5.2   Indirect Treatment 50
4.6   Treatment Examples 51

5   Patterns of Facilitation 57

6   The Scapula and Pelvis 63
6.1   Introduction 63
6.2   Applications 63
6.3   Basic Procedures 64
6.4   Scapular Diagonals 67
6.4.1   Specific Scapular Patterns 67
6.4.2   Specific Uses for Scapular Patterns 74
6.5   Pelvic Diagonals 76
6.5.1   Specific Pelvic Patterns 76
6.5.2   Specific Uses for Pelvic Patterns 88
6.6   Symmetrical, Reciprocal
        and Asymmetrical Exercises 89
6.6.1   Symmetrical-Reciprocal Exercise 89
6.6.2   Asymmetrical Exercise 91

7   The Upper Extremity 93
7.1   Introduction and Basic Procedures 93
7.2   Flexion–Abduction–External Rotation 97
7.2.1   Flexion–Abduction–External Rotation
        with Elbow Flexion 101
7.2.2   Flexion–Abduction–External Rotation
        with Elbow Extension 106
7.3   Extension–Adduction–Internal Rotation 109
7.3.1   Extension–Adduction–Internal Rotation
        with Elbow Extension 112
7.3.2   Extension–Adduction–Internal Rotation
        with Elbow Flexion 115
7.4   Flexion–Adduction–External Rotation 119
7.4.1   Flexion–Adduction–External Rotation
        with Elbow Flexion 122
7.4.2   Flexion–Adduction–External Rotation
        with Elbow Extension 125

7.5	Extension–Abduction–Internal Rotation	129
7.5.1	Extension–Abduction–Internal Rotation with Elbow Extension	133
7.5.2	Extension–Abduction–Internal Rotation with Elbow Flexion	137
7.6	Thrust and Withdrawal Patterns	141
7.6.1	Ulnar Thrust and Withdrawal	143
7.6.2	Radial Thrust and Withdrawal	145
7.7	Bilateral Arm Patterns	147
7.8	Changing the Patient's Position	150
7.8.1	Arm Patterns in a Side Lying Position	150
7.8.2	Arm Patterns Lying Prone on Elbows	151
7.8.3	Arm Patterns in a Sitting Position	152
7.8.4	Arm Patterns in the Quadruped Position	153
7.8.5	Arm Patterns in a Kneeling Position	154
8	**The Lower Extremity**	**155**
8.1	Introduction and Basic Procedures	155
8.2	Flexion–Abduction–Internal Rotation	159
8.2.1	Flexion–Abduction–Internal Rotation with Knee Flexion	162
8.2.2	Flexion–Abduction–Internal Rotation with Knee Extension	165
8.3	Extension–Adduction–External Rotation	169
8.3.1	Extension–Adduction–External Rotation with Knee Extension	174
8.3.2	Extension–Adduction–External Rotation with Knee Flexion	177
8.4	Flexion–Adduction–External Rotation	180
8.4.1	Flexion–Adduction–External Rotation with Knee Flexion	184
8.4.2	Flexion–Adduction–External Rotation with Knee Extension	187
8.5	Extension–Abduction–Internal Rotation	190
8.5.1	Extension–Abduction–Internal Rotation with Knee Extension	193
8.5.2	Extension–Abduction–Internal Rotation with Knee Flexion	196
8.6	Bilateral Leg Patterns	199
8.7	Changing the Patient's Position	203
8.7.1	Leg Patterns in a Sitting Position	203
8.7.2	Leg Patterns in a Prone Position	205
8.7.3	Leg Patterns in a Side Lying Position	207
8.7.4	Leg Patterns in a Quadruped Position	208
8.7.5	Leg Patterns in a Standing Position	210

9   **The Neck** 211
9.1   Introduction and Basic Procedures 211
9.2   Indications 214
9.3   Flexion to the Left, Extension to the Right 215
9.3.1   Flexion/Left Lateral Flexion/Left Rotation 215
9.3.2   Extension/Right Lateral Flexion/Right Rotation .. 219
9.4   Neck for Trunk 221
9.4.1   Neck for Trunk Flexion and Extension 222
9.4.2   Neck for Trunk Lateral Flexion 223

10   **The Trunk** 227
10.1   Introduction and Basic Procedures 227
10.2   Chopping and Lifting 230
10.2.1   Chopping 230
10.2.2   Lifting 234
10.3   Bilateral Leg Patterns for the Trunk 238
10.3.1   Bilateral Lower Extremity Flexion, with Knee
           Flexion, for Lower Trunk Flexion (Right) 238
10.3.2   Bilateral Lower Extremity Extension, with Knee
           Extension, for Lower Trunk Extension (Left) 242
10.3.3   Trunk Lateral Flexion 246
10.4   Combining Patterns for the Trunk 249

11   **Mat Activities** 253
11.1   Introduction: Why Do Mat Activities? 253
11.2   Treatment Goals 254
11.3   Basic Procedures 254
11.4   Techniques 254
11.5   Mat Activities 255
11.5.1   Rolling 255
11.5.2   Prone on Elbows (Forearm Support) 268
11.5.3   Side-Sitting 272
11.5.4   Quadruped 278
11.5.5   Kneeling 286
11.5.6   Half-Kneeling 292
11.5.7   From Hands-and-Feet Position (Arched
           Position on All Fours) to Standing Position
           and Back to Hands-and-Feet Position 295
11.5.8   Exercise in a Sitting Position 296
11.5.9   Bridging 303
11.6   Patient Cases in Mat Activities 308

12   **Gait Training** 319
12.1   The Importance of Walking 319
12.2   Introduction: Basics of Normal Gait 319
12.2.1   The Gait Cycle 319

12.2.2   Trunk and Lower Extremity Joint Motion
          in Normal Gait   320
12.2.3   Muscle Activity During Normal Gait   323
12.3   Gait Analysis: Observation and Manual
          Evaluation   324
12.4   The Theory of Gait Training   327
12.5   The Procedures of Gait Training   327
12.5.1   Approximation and Stretch   328
12.5.2   Using Approximation and Stretch Reflex   329
12.6   Practical Gait Training   331
12.6.1   Preparatory Phase   331
12.6.2   Standing Up and Sitting Down   338
12.6.3   Standing   341
12.6.4   Walking   348
12.6.5   Other Activities   353
12.7   Patient Cases in Gait Training   357

13   **Vital Functions**   365
13.1   Introduction   365
13.1.1   Stimulation and Facilitation   365
13.2   Facial Muscles   365
13.3   Tongue Movements   382
13.4   Swallowing   383
13.5   Speech Disorders   384
13.6   Breathing   385

14   **Activities of Daily Living**   391

15   **Glossary**   397

1 Introduction to Proprioceptive Neuromuscular Facilitation

❏ **Definition.**

Proprioceptive: Having to do with any of the sensory receptors that give information concerning movement and position of the body

Neuromuscular: Involving the nerves and muscles

Facilitation: Making easier

Proprioceptive Neuromuscular Facilitation (PNF) is a concept of treatment. Its underlying philosophy is that all human beings, including those with disabilities, have untapped existing potential (Kabat 1950).

In keeping with this philosophy, there are certain principles that are basic to PNF:

- PNF is an integrated approach: each treatment is directed at a *total human being*, not just at a specific problem or body segment.
- The treatment approach is always *positive*, reinforcing and using that which the patient can do, on a physical and psychological level.
- The primary goal of all treatment is to help patients achieve their *highest level of function*.

This positive functional approach is, we feel, the best way to stimulate patients and to attain superior results from treatment.

This book covers the procedures, techniques, and patterns within PNF. Their application to patient treatment is discussed throughout with special attention to mat activities, gait, and self-care. The emphasis within this book is twofold: developing an understanding of the principles that underlie PNF, and showing through pictures rather than with words how to perform the patterns and activities. Skill in applying the principles and practices of PNF to patient treatment cannot be learned only from a book. We recommend that the learner combines reading with classroom practice and patient treatment under the supervision of a skilled PNF practitioner.

The aims of this book are:

- To show the PNF method and, in so doing, help students and practitioners of physical therapy in their PNF training.
- To attain a uniformity in practical treatment.
- To record the most recent developments in PNF and put them into word and picture.

Basic *neurophysiologic* principles:

The work of Sir Charles Sherrington was important in the development of the procedures and techniques of PNF. The following useful definitions were abstracted from his work (Sherrington 1947):

- *Afterdischarge*: The effect of a stimulus continues after the stimulus stops. If the strength and duration of the stimulus increase, the afterdischarge increases also. The feeling of increased power that comes after a maintained static contraction is a result of afterdischarge.
- *Temporal summation*: A succession of weak stimuli (subliminal) occurring within a certain (short) period of time combine (summate) to cause excitation.
- *Spatial summation*: Weak stimuli applied simultaneously to different areas of the body reinforce each other (summate) to cause excitation. Temporal and spatial summation can combine for greater activity.
- *Irradiation*: This is a spreading and increased strength of a response. It occurs when either the number of stimuli or the strength of the stimuli is increased. The response may be either excitation or inhibition.
- *Successive induction*: An increased excitation of the agonist muscles follows stimulation (contraction) of their antagonists. Techniques involving reversal of antagonists make use of this property (Induction: stimulation, increased excitability.).
- *Reciprocal innervation* (reciprocal inhibition): Contraction of muscles is accompanied by simultaneous inhibition of their antagonists. Reciprocal innervation is a necessary part of coordinated motion. Relaxation techniques make use of this property.

**"The nervous system is continuous throughout its extent –
there are no isolated parts."**

References

Kabat H (1950) Studies on neuromuscular dysfunction. XIII. New concepts and techniques of neuromuscular reeducation for paralysis. Perm Found Med Bull 8 (3):121–143

Sherrington C (1947) The integrative action of the nervous system. Yale University Press, New Haven

2 Basic Procedures for Facilitation

THERAPEUTIC GOALS

The basic facilitation procedures provide tools for the therapist to help the patient gain efficient motor function and increased motor control. Their effectiveness does not depend on having the conscious cooperation of the patient. These basic procedures are used to:
- Increase the patient's ability to move or remain stable.
- Guide the motion by proper grips and appropriate resistance.
- Help the patient achieve coordinated motion through timing.
- Increase the patient's stamina and avoid fatigue.

The basic facilitation procedures overlap in their effects. For example, **resistance** is necessary to make the **stretch reflex** effective (Gellhorn 1949). The effect of resistance changes with the alignment of the therapist's body and the direction of the manual contact. The timing of these procedures is important to get an optimal response from the patient. For example, a preparatory verbal command comes before the stretch reflex. Changing of the manual contacts should be timed to cue the patient for a change in the direction of motion.

We can use these basic procedures to treat patients with *any diagnosis or condition*, although a patient's condition may rule out the use of some of them. The therapist should avoid causing or increasing pain. Pain is an inhibitor of effective and coordinated muscular performance and it can be a sign of potential harm (Hislop 1960; Fisher 1967). Other contraindications are mainly common sense: for example, not using approximation on an extremity with an unhealed fracture. In the presence of unstable joints, the therapist should take great care when using traction or the stretch reflex.

The *basic procedures* for facilitation are:
- **Resistance**: To aid muscle contraction and motor control, to increase strength, aid motor learning.
- **Irradiation and reinforcement**: Use of the spread of the response to stimulation.
- **Manual contact**: To increase power and guide motion with grip and pressure.
- **Body position and body mechanics**: Guidance and control of motion or stability.

- **Verbal** (commands): Use of words and the appropriate vocal volume to direct the patient.
- **Vision:** Use of vision to guide motion and increase force.
- **Traction or approximation:** The elongation or compression of the limbs and trunk to facilitate motion and stability.
- **Stretch:** The use of muscle elongation and the stretch reflex to facilitate contraction and decrease muscle fatigue.
- **Timing:** Promote normal timing and increase muscle contraction through "timing for emphasis".
- **Patterns:** Synergistic mass movements, components of functional normal motion.

Combine these basic procedures to get a maximal response from the patient.

2.1 Resistance

THERAPEUTIC GOALS ■■■■■■■■■■■■■■■■■■■■■■■■■■■■■■■■■■

Resistance is used in treatment to:
- Facilitate the ability of the muscle to contract.
- Increase motor control and motor learning.
- Help the patient gain an awareness of motion and its direction.
- Increase strength.

Most of the PNF techniques evolved from knowing the effects of resistance.

❑ **Definition.** The amount of resistance provided during an activity must be correct for the patient's condition and the goal of the activity. This we call *optimal resistance*.

Gellhorn showed that when a muscle contraction is resisted, that muscle's response to cortical stimulation increases. The active muscle tension produced by resistance is the *most effective* proprioceptive facilitation. The magnitude of that facilitation is related directly to the amount of resistance (Gellhorn 1949; Loofbourrow and Gellhorn 1949). Proprioceptive reflexes from contracting muscles increase the response of synergistic muscles[1] at the same joint and associated synergists at neighboring joints. This facilitation can spread from proximal to distal and from distal to proximal. Antagonists of the facilitated muscles are usually inhibited. If the muscle activity in the agonists becomes intense, there may be activity in the antagonistic muscle groups as well (co-contraction). (Gellhorn 1947; Loofbourrow and Gellhorn 1948).

How we give resistance depends on the kind of muscle contraction being resisted (Fig. 2.1).

---

[1] Synergists are muscles which act with other muscles to produce coordinated motion.

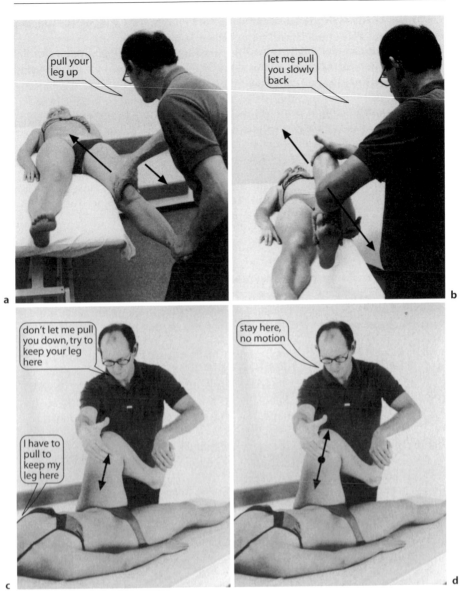

Fig. 2.1 a–d. Types of muscle contraction of the patient. **a** Isotonic concentric: movement into a shortened range; the force or resistance provided by the patient is stronger. **b** Isotonic eccentric: the force or resistance provided by the therapist is stronger; movement into the lengthened range. **c** Stabilizing isotonic: the patient tries to move but is prevented by the therapist or another outside force; the forces exerted by both are the same. **d** Isometric (static): the intent of both the patient and the therapist is that no motion occurs; the forces exerted by both are the same

❏ **Definition.** We define the *types of muscle contraction* as follows (International PNF Association, unpublished handout):
- *Isotonic* (dynamic): The intent of the patient is to produce motion.
  - ▶ Concentric: Shortening of the agonist produces motion.
  - ▶ Eccentric: An outside force, gravity or resistance, produces the motion. The motion is restrained by the controlled lengthening of the agonist.
  - ▶ Stabilizing isotonic: The intent of the patient is motion; the motion is prevented by an outside force (usually resistance).
- *Isometric* (static): The intent of both the patient and the therapist is that no motion occurs.

The resistance to concentric or eccentric muscle contractions should be adjusted so that motion can occur in a smooth and coordinated manner. Resistance to a stabilizing contraction must be controlled to maintain the stabilized position. When resisting an isometric contraction, the resistance should be increased and decreased gradually so that no motion occurs.

It is important that the resistance does not cause pain or unwanted fatigue. Both the therapist and the patient should avoid breath-holding. Timed and controlled inhalations and exhalations can increase the patient's strength and active range of motion.

2.2 Irradiation and Reinforcement

Properly applied resistance results in irradiation and reinforcement.

❏ **Irradiation.** We define *irradiation* as the spread of the response to stimulation.

This response can be seen as increased facilitation (contraction) or inhibition (relaxation) in the synergistic muscles and patterns of movement. The response increases as the stimuli increase in intensity or duration (Sherrington 1947). Kabat (1961) wrote that it is resistance to motion that produces irradiation, and the spread of the muscular activity will occur in specific patterns.

❏ **Reinforcement.** *Reinforce*, as defined in Webster's Ninth New Collegiate Dictionary, is "to strengthen by fresh addition, make stronger."
The therapist directs the reinforcement of the weaker muscles by the amount of resistance given to the strong muscles.

Increasing the amount of resistance will increase the amount and extent of the muscular response. Changing the movement that is resisted or the position of the patient will also change the results. The therapist adjusts the amount of resistance and type of muscle contraction to suit 1) the condition of the patient, and 2) the goal of the treatment. Because each patient reacts differently, it is not possible to give general instructions on how much resistance to give or which movements to resist. By assessing the results of the treatment, the therapist can determine the best uses of resistance, irradiation, and reinforcement.

THERAPEUTIC GOALS ▰▰▰▰

Examples of the use of resistance in patient treatment:
- Resist muscle contractions in a sound limb to produce contraction of the muscles in the immobilized contralateral limb.
- Resist hip flexion to cause contraction of the trunk flexor muscles (Fig. 2.2).
- Resist supination of the forearm to facilitate contraction of the external rotators of that shoulder.
- Resist hip flexion with adduction and external rotation to facilitate the ipsilateral dorsiflexor muscles to contract with inversion (Fig. 2.3).
- Resist neck flexion to stimulate trunk and hip flexion. Resist neck extension to stimulate trunk and hip extension.

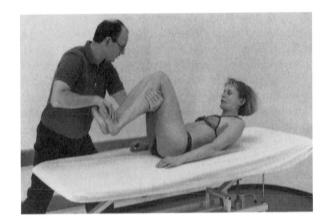

Fig. 2.2. Irradiation into the trunk flexor muscles when doing bilateral leg patterns

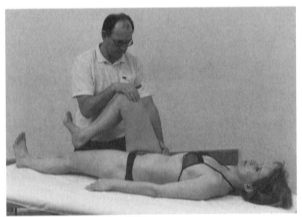

Fig. 2.3. Irradiation to dorsiflexion and inversion with the leg pattern flexion–adduction–external rotation

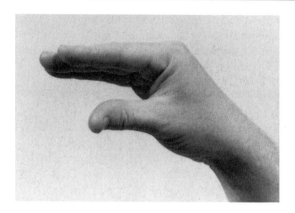

Fig. 2.4. The lumbrical grip

2.3 Manual Contact

THERAPEUTIC GOALS ▬▬▬▬▬▬▬

- Pressure on a muscle to aid that muscle's ability to contract.
- Pressure that is opposite to the direction of motion on any point of a moving limb stimulate the synergistic limb muscles to reinforce the movement.
- Contact on the patient's trunk to help the limb motion indirectly by promoting trunk stability.

The therapist's grip stimulates the patient's *skin receptors* and other pressure receptors. This contact gives the patient information about the proper direction of motion. The therapist's hand should be placed to apply the pressure opposite the direction of motion. The sides of the arm or leg are considered neutral surfaces and may be held.

To control movement and resist rotation the therapist uses a *lumbrical grip* (Fig. 2.4). In this grip the pressure comes from flexion at the metacarpophalangeal joints, allowing the therapist's fingers to conform to the body part. The lumbrical grip gives the therapist good control of the three-dimensional motion without causing the patient pain due to squeezing or putting too much pressure on bony body parts (Fig. 2.5).

2.4 Body Position and Body Mechanics

THERAPEUTIC GOALS ▬▬▬▬▬▬▬

- Give the therapist effective control of the patient's motion.
- Facilitate control of the direction of the resistance.
- Enable the therapist to give resistance without fatiguing.

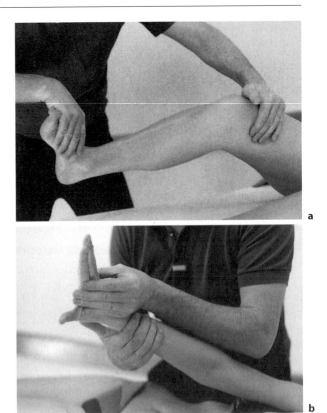

Fig. 2.5 a, b. Lumbrical grips. **a** For the leg pattern flexion–adduction–external rotation. **b** For the arm pattern flexion–abduction–external rotation

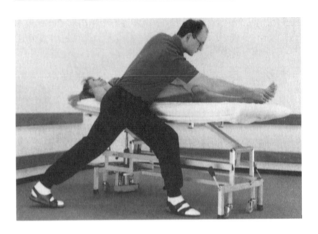

Fig. 2.6. Positioning of the therapist's body for the leg pattern flexion–abduction–internal rotation

Johnson and Saliba first developed the material on body position presented here. They observed that more effective control of the patient's motion came when the therapist was in the line of the desired motion. As the therapist shifted position, the direction of the resistance changed and the patient's movement changed with it. From this knowledge they developed the following guidelines for the therapist's body position (G. Johnson and V. Saliba, unpublished handout 1985):

- The therapist's body should be *in line* with the desired motion or force. To line up properly, the therapist's shoulders and pelvis face the direction of the motion. The arms and hands also line up with the motion. If the therapist cannot keep the proper body position, the hands and arms maintain alignment with the motion (Fig. 2.6).
- The resistance comes from the therapist's *body* while the hands and arms stay comparatively relaxed. By using body weight the therapist can give prolonged resistance without fatiguing. The relaxed hands allow the therapist to feel the patient's responses.

2.5 Verbal Stimulation (Commands)

THERAPEUTIC GOALS ■■

- Guide the start of movement or the muscle contractions.
- Affect the strength of the resulting muscle contractions.
- Give the patient corrections.

The verbal command tells the patient what to do and when to do it. The therapist must always bear in mind that the command is given to the patient, not to the body part being treated. Preparatory instructions need to be clear and concise, without unnecessary words. They may be combined with passive motion to teach the desired movement.

The *timing* of the command is important to coordinate the patient's reactions with the therapist's hands and resistance. It guides the start of movement and muscle contractions. It helps give the patient corrections for motion or stability.

Timing of the command is also very important when using the stretch reflex. The initial command should come immediately before the stretch reflex to coordinate the patient's conscious effort with the reflex response (Evarts and Tannji 1974). The action command is repeated to urge greater effort or redirect the motion.

The *volume* with which the command is given can affect the strength of the resulting muscle contractions (Johansson et al. 1983). The therapist should give a louder command when a strong muscle contraction is desired and use a softer and calmer tone when the goal is relaxation or relief of pain.

The command is divided into three parts:
1. *Preparation*: readies the patient for action
2. *Action*: tells the patient to start the action
3. *Correction*: tells the patient how to correct and modify the action

For example, the command for the lower extremity pattern of flexion–adduction–external rotation with knee flexion might be [preparation] "ready, and"; [action] "now pull your leg up and in"; [correction] "keep pulling your toes up" (to correct lack of dorsiflexion).

2.6 Vision

THERAPEUTIC GOALS
- Promote a more powerful muscle contraction.
- Help the patient control and correct position and motion.
- Influence both the head and body motion.
- Provide an avenue of communication and help to ensure cooperative interaction.

The feedback from the visual sensory system can promote a more powerful muscle contraction. For example, when a patient looks at his or her arm or leg while exercising it, a stronger contraction is achieved. Using vision helps the patient control and correct his or her position and motion.

Moving the eyes will influence both the *head and body motion*. For example, when patients looks in the direction they want to move, the head follows the eye motion. The head motion in turn will facilitate larger and stronger trunk motion (Fig. 2.7).

Eye contact between patient and therapist provides another avenue of communication and helps to ensure cooperative interaction.

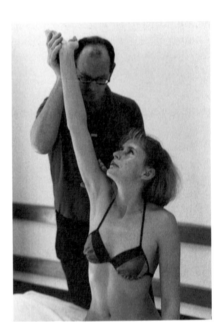

Fig. 2.7. Visual control

2.7 Traction and Approximation

❏ Definition.

Traction is the elongation of the trunk or an extremity.

Knott, Voss, and their colleagues theorized that the therapeutic effects of traction are due to stimulation of receptors in the joints (Knott and Voss 1968; Voss et al. 1985). Traction also acts as a stretch stimulus by elongating the muscles.

Apply the traction force gradually until the desired result is achieved. The traction is maintained throughout the movement and combined with appropriate resistance.

THERAPEUTIC GOALS ▬▬▬▬▬▬▬▬▬▬▬▬

Traction is used to:
- Facilitate motion, especially pulling and antigravity motions.
- Aid in elongation of muscle tissue when using the stretch reflex.
- Resist some part of the motion. For example, use traction at the beginning of shoulder flexion to resist scapula elevation.

Traction of the affected part is helpful when treating patients with joint pain.

❏ Definition.

Approximation is the compression of the trunk or an extremity.

The muscle contractions following the approximation are thought to be due to stimulation of joint receptors (Knott and Voss 1968; Voss et al. 1985). Another possible reason for the increased muscular response is to counteract the disturbance of position or posture caused by the approximation. Given gradually and gently, approximation may aid in the treatment of painful and unstable joints.

THERAPEUTIC GOALS ▬▬▬▬▬▬▬▬▬▬▬▬

Approximation is used to:
- Promote stabilization
- Facilitate weight-bearing and the contraction of antigravity muscles
- Facilitate upright reactions
- Resist some component of motion. For example, use approximation at the end of shoulder flexion to resist scapula elevation.

There are two ways to apply the approximation:
- *Quick* approximation: the force is applied quickly to elicit a reflex-type response.
- *Slow* approximation: the force is applied gradually up to the patient's tolerance.

The approximation force is always maintained, whether the approximation is done quickly or slowly. The therapist maintains the force and gives resistance to the resulting muscular response. An appropriate command should be coordinated with the application of the approximation, for example "hold it" or "stand tall." The patient's joints should be properly aligned and in a weight-bearing position before the approximation is given.

When the therapist feels that the active muscle contraction decreases the approximation is repeated and resistance given.

2.8 Stretch

❏ *Stretch stimulus.*

THERAPEUTIC GOALS ▬▬▬▬▬▬▬▬▬▬▬▬▬▬▬▬▬▬▬▬
* Facilitate muscle contractions.
* Facilitate contraction of associated synergistic muscles.

The *stretch stimulus* occurs when a muscle is *elongated*. Stretch stimulus is used during normal activities as a preparatory motion to facilitate the muscle contractions. The stimulus facilitates the elongated muscle, synergistic muscles at the same joint, and other associated synergistic muscles (Loofbourrow and Gellhorn 1948). Greater facilitation comes from lengthening all the *synergistic muscles* of a limb or the trunk. For example, elongation of the anterior tibial muscle facilitates that muscle and also facilitates the hip flexor–adductor–external rotator muscle group. If just the hip flexor–adductor–external rotator muscle group is elongated, the hip muscles and the anterior tibial muscle share the increased facilitation. If all the muscles of the hip and ankle are lengthened simultaneously, the excitability in those limb muscles increases further and spreads to the synergistic trunk flexor muscles.

❏ *Stretch reflex.*

THERAPEUTIC GOALS ▬▬▬▬▬▬▬▬▬▬▬▬▬▬▬▬▬▬▬▬
How, why, and when to use the stretch reflex is described in Chapter III, Sect. 3.4.

The *stretch reflex* is elicited from muscles that are under tension, either from elongation or from contraction. The reflex has *two parts*. The *first* is a short-latency spinal reflex that produces little force and may not be of functional significance. The *second* part, called the functional stretch response, has a longer latency but produces a more powerful and functional contraction (Conrad and Meyer-Lohmann 1980; Chan 1984). To be effective as a treatment, the muscular contraction following the stretch must be resisted.

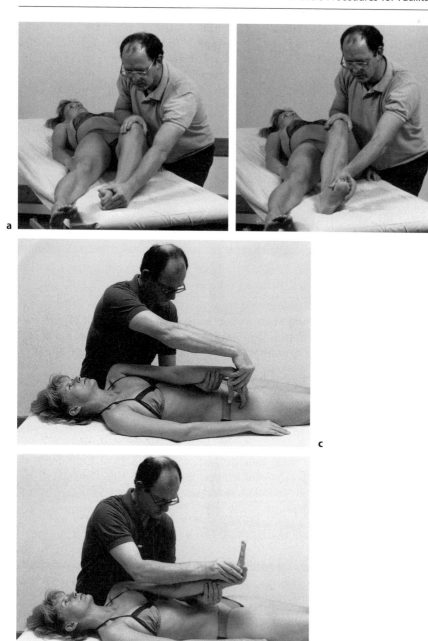

Fig. 2.8 a–d. Timing for emphasis by preventing motion. **a, b** Leg pattern flexion–abduction–internal rotation with knee flexion. The strong motions of the hip and knee are blocked and the dorsiflexion–eversion of the ankle exercised using repeated stretch reflex. **c, d** Arm pattern flexion–abduction–external rotation. The stronger shoulder motions are blocked while exercising radial extension of the wrist

The strength of the muscular contraction produced by the stretch is affected by the intent of the subject, and therefore, by prior instruction. Monkeys show changes in their motor cortex and stronger responses when they are instructed to resist the stretch. The same increase in response has been shown to happen in humans when they are told to resist a muscle stretch (Hammond 1956; Evarts and Tannji 1974; Chan 1984).

2.9 Timing

THERAPEUTIC GOALS ▮▬▬▬▬▬▬▬▬▬▬▬▬▬▬▬▬▬▬▬▬▬▬▬

- Normal timing provides continuous, coordinated motion until a task is accomplished.
- Timing for emphasis redirects the energy of a strong contraction into weaker muscles.

❏ Definition.
Timing is the sequencing of motions.

Normal movement requires a smooth sequence of activity, and coordinated movement requires precise timing of that sequence. Functional movement requires continuous, coordinated motion until the task is accomplished.

❏ Definition.
Normal timing of most coordinated and efficient motions is from distal to proximal.

The evolution of control and coordination during development proceeds from cranial to caudal and from proximal to distal (Jacobs 1967). In infancy the arm determines where the hand goes, but after the grasp matures the hand directs the course of the arm movements (Halvorson 1931). The small motions that adults use to maintain standing balance proceed from distal (ankle) to proximal (hip and trunk) (Nashner 1977). To restore normal timing of motion may become a goal of the treatment.

❏ Definition.
Timing for emphasis involves changing the normal sequencing of motions to emphasize a particular muscle or a desired activity.

Kabat (1947) wrote that prevention of motion in a stronger synergist will redirect the energy of that contraction into a weaker muscle. This alteration of timing stimulates the proprioceptive reflexes in the muscles by resistance and stretch. The best results come when the strong muscles score at least "good" in strength (Manual Muscle Test grade 4; Partridge 1954).

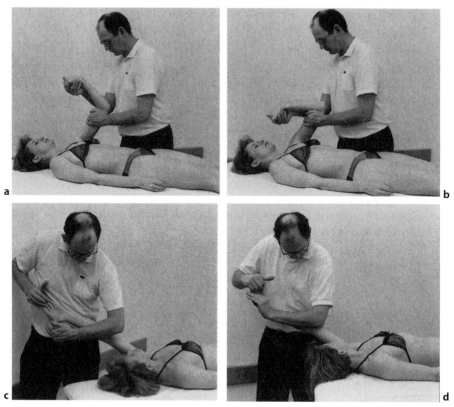

Fig. 2.9 a–d. Timing for emphasis using stabilizing contractions of strong muscles. **a,b** Exercising elbow flexion using the pattern of flexion–adduction–external rotation with stabilizing contractions of the strong shoulder and wrist muscles. **c,d** Exercising finger flexion using the pattern extension–adduction–internal rotation with stabilizing contraction of the strong shoulder muscles

There are two ways the therapist can alter the normal timing for therapeutic purposes (Figs. 2.8, 2.9):

- By preventing all the motions of a pattern except the one that is to be emphasized.
- By resisting an isometric or maintained contraction of the strong motions in a pattern while exercising the weaker muscles. This resistance to the static contraction locks in that segment, so resisting the contraction is called "locking it in."

2.10 Patterns

The patterns of facilitation may be considered one of the basic procedures of PNF. For greater clarity we discuss and illustrate them in Chapter 5.

References

Chan CWY (1984) Neurophysiological basis underlying the use of resistance to facilitate movement. Physiother Can 36 (6):335–341

Conrad B, Meyer-Lohmann J (1980) The long-loop transcortical load compensating reflex. Trends Neurosci 3:269–272

Evarts EV, Tannji J (1974) Gating of motor cortex reflexes by prior instruction. Brain Res 71:479–494

Fischer E (1967) Factors affecting motor learning. Am J Phys Med Rehabil 46 (1):511–519

Gellhorn E (1947) Patterns of muscular activity in man. Arch Phys Med Rehabil 28:568–574

Gellhorn E (1949) Proprioception and the motor cortex. Brain 72:35–62

Halvorson HM (1931) An experimental study of prehension in infants by means of systematic cinema records. Genet Psychol Monogr 10:279–289. Reprinted in: Jacobs MJ (1967) Development of normal motor behavior. Am J Phys Med Rehabil 46 (1):41–51

Hammond PH (1956) The influences of prior instruction to the subject on an apparently involuntary neuromuscular response. J Physiol (Lond) 132:17P–18P

Hislop HH (1960) Pain and exercise. Phys Ther Rev 40 (2):98–106

Jacobs MJ (1967) Development of normal motor behavior. Am J Phys Med Rehabil 46 (1):41–51

Johansson CA, Kent BE, Shepard KF (1983) Relationship between verbal command volume and magnitude of muscle contraction. Phys Ther 63 (8):1260–1265

Kabat H (1947) Studies on neuromuscular dysfunction, XI: New principles of neuromuscular reeducation. Perm Found Med Bull 5 (3):111–123

Kabat H (1961) Proprioceptive facilitation in therapeutic exercise. In: Licht S Johnson EW (eds) Therapeutic exercise, 2nd edn. Waverly, Baltimore

Knott M, Voss DE (1968) Proprioceptive neuromuscular facilitation: patterns and techniques, 2nd edn. Harper and Row, New York

Loofbourrow GN, Gellhorn E (1948) Proprioceptively induced reflex patterns. Am J Physiol 154:433–438

Loofbourrow GN, Gellhorn E (1949) Proprioceptive modification of reflex patterns. J Neurophysiol 12:435–446

Nashner LM (1977) Fixed patterns of rapid postural responses among leg muscles during stance. Exp Brain Res 30:13–24

Partridge MJ (1954) Electromyographic demonstration of facilitation. Phys Ther Rev 34 (5):227–233

Sherrington C (1947) The integrative action of the nervous system, 2nd edn. Yale University Press, New Haven

Voss DE, Ionta M, Meyers B (1985) Proprioceptive neuromuscular facilitation: patterns and techniques, 3rd edn. Harper and Row, New York

Webster's Ninth New Collegiate Dictionary (1984) Merriam-Webster, Springfield

Further Reading

General

Griffin JW (1974) Use of proprioceptive stimuli in therapeutic exercise. Phys Ther 54 (10):1072–1079

Payton OD, Hirt S, Newton RA (eds) (1977) Scientific basis for neuro-physiologic approaches to therapeutic exercise: an anthology. Davis, Philadelphia

Resistance, Irradiation and Reinforcement

Hellebrandt FA (1958) Application of the overload principle to muscle training in man. Arch Phys Med Rehabil 37:278–283

Hellebrandt FA, Houtz SJ (1956) Mechanisms of muscle training in man: experimental demonstration of the overload principle. Phys Ther 36 (6):371–383

Hellebrandt FA, Houtz SJ (1958) Methods of muscle training: the influence of pacing. Phys Ther 38:319–322

Hellebrandt FA, Waterland JC (1962) Expansion of motor patterning under exercise stress. Am J Phys Med Rehabil 41:56–66

Moore JC (1975) Excitation overflow: an electromyographic investigation. Arch Phys Med Rehabil 56:115–120

Stretch

Burg D, Szumski AJ, Struppler A, Velho F (1974) Assessment of fusimotor contribution to reflex reinforcement in humans. J Neurol Neurosurg Psychiatry 37:1012–1021

Cavagna GA, Dusman B, Margaria R (1968) Positive work done by a previously stretched muscle. J Appl Physiol 24 (1):21–32

Chan CWY, Kearney RE (1982) Is the functional stretch response servo controlled or preprogrammed? Electroencephalogr Clin Neurophysiol 53:310–324

Ghez C, Shinoda Y (1978) Spinal mechanisms of the functional stretch reflex. Exp Brain Res 32:55–68

3 Techniques

Introduction

The goal of the PNF techniques is to promote functional movement through facilitation, inhibition, strengthening, and relaxation of muscle groups. The techniques use concentric, eccentric, and static muscle contractions. These muscle contractions with properly graded resistance and suitable facilitatory procedures are combined and adjusted to fit the needs of each patient.

- To increase the range of motion and strengthen the muscles in the newly gained range of motion. Use a relaxation technique such as Contract-Relax to increase range of motion. Follow with a facilitatory technique such as Dynamic Reversals (Slow Reversals) or Combination of Isotonics to increase the strength and control in the newly gained range of motion.
- To relieve muscle fatigue during strengthening exercises. After using a strengthening technique such as Repeated Stretch (repeated stretch reflex), go immediately into Dynamic Reversals (Slow Reversals) to relieve fatigue in the exercised muscles. The repeated stretch reflex permits muscles to work longer without fatiguing. Alternating contractions of the antagonistic muscles relieves the fatigue that follows repeated exercise of one group of muscles.

We have grouped the PNF techniques so that those with similar functions or actions are together. Where new terminology is used, the name describes the activity or type of muscle contraction involved. When the terminology differs from that used by Knott and Voss (1968), both names are given.

For example, Reversal of Antagonists is a general class of techniques in which the patient first contracts the agonistic muscles then contracts their antagonists without pause or relaxation. Within that class, Dynamic Reversal of Antagonist is an isotonic technique where the patient first moves in one direction and then in the opposite without stopping. Rhythmic Stabilization involves isometric contractions of the antagonistic muscle groups. In this technique, motion is not intended by either the patient or the therapist. We use both reversal techniques to increase strength and range of motion.

Rhythmic Stabilization works to increase the patient's ability to stabilize or hold a position as well.[1]

The techniques described are:
- Rhythmic Initiation
- Combination of Isotonics (G. Johnson and V. Saliba, unpublished handout 1988) (also called Reversal of Agonists; Sullivan et al. 1982)
- Reversal of Antagonists
  - ▶ Dynamic Reversal of Antagonists (incorporates Slow Reversal)
  - ▶ Stabilizing Reversal
  - ▶ Rhythmic Stabilization
- Repeated Stretch (Repeated Contraction)
  - ▶ Repeated Stretch from beginning of range
  - ▶ Repeated Stretch through range
- Contract-Relax
- Hold-Relax
- Replication

In presenting each technique we give a short characterization, the goals, uses, and any contraindications. Following are full descriptions of each technique, examples, and ways in which they may be modified.

3.1 Rhythmic Initiation

Characterization

Rhythmic motion of the limb or body through the desired range, starting with passive motion and progressing to active resisted movement.

Goals

- Aid in initiation of motion
- Improve coordination and sense of motion
- Normalize the rate of motion, either increasing or decreasing it
- Teach the motion
- Help the patient to relax

---

[1] G. Johnson and V. Saliba were the first to use the terms "stabilizing reversal of antagonists," "dynamic reversal of antagonist," "combination of isotonics," and "repeated stretch" in an unpublished course handout at the Institute of Physical Art (1979).

Indications

- Difficulties in initiating motion
- Movement too slow or too fast
- Uncoordinated or dysrhythmic motion
- General tension

Description

- The therapist starts by moving the patient passively through the range of motion, using the speed of the verbal command to set the rhythm.
- The patient is asked to begin working actively in the desired direction. The return motion is done by the therapist.
- The therapist resists the active movement, maintaining the rhythm with the verbal commands.
- To finish the patient should make the motion independently.

Example: Trunk extension in a sitting position:
▶ Move the patient passively from trunk flexion into extension and then back to the flexed position. "Let me move you up straight. Good, now let me move you back down and then up again."
▶ When the patient is relaxed and moving easily, ask for active assisted motion. "Help me a little coming up straight. Now relax and let me bring you forward."
▶ Then begin resisting the motion. "Push up straight. Let me bring you forward. Now push up straight again."
▶ Independent: "Now straighten up on your own."

Modifications

- The technique can be finished by using eccentric as well as concentric muscle contractions (Combination of Isotonics).
- The technique may be finished with active motion in both directions (Reversal of Antagonists).

→ **Points to remember:**
- **Use the speed of the verbal command to set the rhythm.**
- **At the end the patient should make the motion independently.**
- **The technique may be combined with other techniques.**

3.2 Combination of Isotonics (described by Gregg Johnson and Vicky Saliba)

Characterization

Combined concentric, eccentric, and stabilizing contractions of one group of muscles (agonists) without relaxation. For treatment, start where the patient has the most strength or best coordination.

Goals

- Active control of motion
- Coordination
- Increase the active range of motion
- Strengthen
- Functional training in eccentric control of movement

Indications

- Decreased eccentric control
- Lack of coordination or ability to move in a desired direction
- Decreased active range of motion
- Lack of active motion within the range of motion

Description

- The therapist resists the patient's moving actively through a desired range of motion (concentric contraction).
- At the end of motion the therapist tells the patient to stay in that position (stabilizing contraction).
- When stability is attained the therapist tells the patient to allow the part to be moved slowly back to the starting position (eccentric contraction).
- There is no relaxation between the different types of muscle activities and the therapist's hands remain on the same surface.

Note: The eccentric or stabilizing muscle contraction may come before the concentric contraction.

Example: Trunk extension in a sitting position (Fig. 3.1 a, b):
▶ Resist the patient's concentric contraction into trunk extension. "Push back away from me."
▶ At the end of the patient's active range of motion, tell the patient to stabilize in that position. "Stop, stay there, don't let me pull you forward."

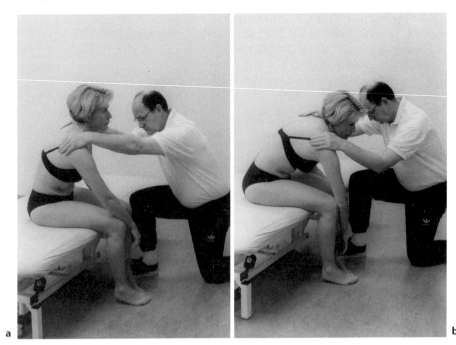

a   b

Fig. 3.1 a,b. Combination of Isotonics: coming forward with eccentric contraction of trunk extensor muscles

▶ After the patient is stable, move the patient back to the original position while he or she maintains control with an eccentric contraction of the trunk extensor muscles. "Now let me pull you forward, but slowly."

Modifications

- The technique may be combined with Reversal of Antagonists.

Example: Trunk flexion combined with trunk extension:
▶ After repeating the above exercise a number of times, tell the patient to move actively with concentric contractions into trunk flexion.
▶ Then you may repeat the exercise with trunk flexion, using Combination of Isotonics, or continue with Reversal of Antagonists for trunk flexion and extension.

Modification

- The technique can start at the end of the range of motion and begin with eccentric contractions.

Example: Eccentric trunk extension in a sitting position (Fig. 3.1 a, b):
▶ Start the exercise with the patient in trunk extension.
▶ Move the patient from extension back to trunk flexion while he or she maintains control with an eccentric contraction of the trunk extension muscles. "Now let me pull you forward, but slowly."

Modifications

- One type of muscle contraction can be changed to another before completing the full range of motion.
- A change can be made from the concentric to the eccentric muscle contraction without stopping or stabilizing.

Example: Trunk flexion in a sitting position:
▶ Resist the patient's concentric contraction into trunk flexion. "Push forward toward me."
▶ After the patient reaches the desired degree of trunk flexion, move the patient back to the original position while he or she maintains control with an eccentric contraction of the trunk flexor muscles. "Now let me push you back, but slowly."

> → **Points to remember**
> - **Start where the patient has the most strength or best coordination**
> - **The stabilizing or eccentric muscle contraction may come first**
> - **To emphasize the end of the range, start there with eccentric contractions**

3.3 Reversal of Antagonists

These techniques are based on Sherrington's principle of successive induction.

3.3.1 Dynamic Reversals (Incorporates Slow Reversal)

Characterization

Active motion changing from one direction (agonist) to the opposite (antagonist) without pause or relaxation. In normal life we often see this kind of muscle activity; throwing a ball, bicycling, walking etc.

Goals

- Increase active range of motion
- Increase strength
- Develop coordination (smooth reversal of motion)
- Prevent or reduce fatigue
- Increase endurance

Indications

- Decreased active range of motion
- Weakness of the agonistic muscles
- Decreased ability to change direction of motion
- Exercised muscles begin to fatigue

Description

- The therapist resists the patient's moving in one direction, usually the stronger or better direction (Fig. 3.2 a).

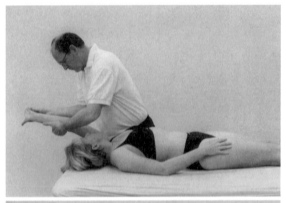

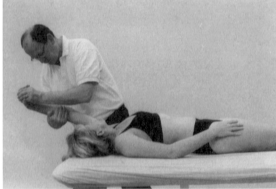

Fig. 3.2 a–b. Dynamic Reversal of the arm diagonal flexion-abduction into extension-adduction. a Reaching the end of flexion-abduction. b After changing the hands, resisting the movement into extension-adduction

- As the end of the desired range of motion approaches the therapist reverses the grip on the distal portion of the moving segment and gives a command to prepare for the change of direction.
- At the end of the desired movement the therapist gives the action command to reverse direction, without relaxation, and gives resistance to the new motion starting with the distal part (Fig. 3.2 b).
- When the patient begins moving in the opposite direction the therapist reverses the proximal grip so all resistance opposes the new direction.
- The reversals may be done as often as necessary.

Normally we start with contraction of the stronger pattern and finish with contraction of the weaker pattern. However, don't leave the patient with a limb "in the air".

Example: Reversing lower extremity motion from flexion to extension:
▶ Resist the desired (stronger) pattern of lower extremity flexion. "Foot up and lift your leg up." (Fig. 3.3 a)
▶ As the patient's leg approaches the end of the range, give a verbal cue (preparatory command) to get the patient's attention while you slide the hand that was resisting on the dorsum of the foot to the plantar surface (the dorsiflexor muscles are still active by irradiation from the proximal grip) to resist the patient's foot during the reverse motion.
▶ When you are ready for the patient to move in the new direction give the action command "Now push your foot down and kick your leg down." (Fig. 3.3 b)
▶ As the patient starts to move in the new direction, move your proximal hand so that it also resists the new direction of motion (Fig. 3.3 c).

Modifications

- Instead of moving through the full range, the change of direction can be used to emphasize a particular range of the motion.
  ▶ Start the reversal from flexion to extension before reaching the end of the flexion motion. You may reverse again before reaching the end of the extension motion:
- The speed used in one or both directions can be varied.
- The technique can begin with small motions in each direction, increasing the range of motion as the patient's skill increases.
- The range of motion can be decreased in each direction until the patient is stabilized in both directions.
- The patient can be instructed to hold his or her position or stabilize at any point in the range of motion or at the end of the range. This can be done before and after reversing direction.

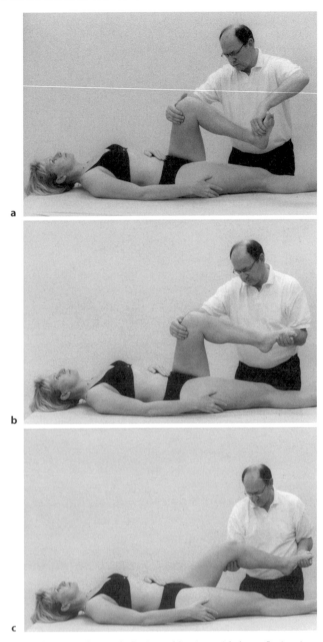

Fig. 3.3 a–c. Dynamic Reversal of the leg diagonal: flexion-adduction with knee flexion into extension-abduction with knee extension. **a** Resisting flexion adduction. **b** Distal grip changed and motion into extension-abduction started. **c** Resisting extension abduction

Example: Reversing lower extremity motion with stabilization before the reversal.

▶ When the patient reaches the end of the flexion motion give a stabilizing command ("keep your leg up there").

▶ After the leg is stabilized change the distal hand and ask for the next motion ("kick down").

Example: Reversing lower extremity motion with stabilization after the reversal.

▶ After changing the distal hand to the plantar surface of the foot give a stabilizing command ("keep your leg there, don't let me push it up any further").

▶ When the leg is stabilized, give a motion command to continue to exercise ("now kick down").

- The technique can begin with the stronger direction to gain irradiation into the weaker muscles after reversing.
- A reversal should be done whenever the agonistic muscles begin to fatigue.
- If increasing strength is the goal the resistance increases with each change and the command asks for more power.

→ **Points to remember**
- Only use an initial stretch reflex. Do not re-stretch when changing the direction because the antagonist muscles are not yet under tension
- Resist, don't assist the patient when changing the direction of motion
- Change the direction to emphasize a particular range of the motion

---

3.3.2 Stabilizing Reversals

Characterization

Alternating isotonic contractions opposed by enough resistance to prevent motion. The command is a dynamic command ("push against my hands", or "don't let me push you") and the therapist allows only a very small movement.

Goals

- Increase stability and balance
- Increase muscle strength
- Increase coordination between agonist and antagonist

Indications

- Decreased stability
- Weakness
- Patient is unable to contract muscle isometrically

Description

- The therapist gives resistance to the patient, starting in the strongest direction, while asking the patient to oppose the force. Very little motion is allowed. Approximation or traction should be used to increase stability.
- When the patient is fully resisting the force the therapist moves one hand and begins to give resistance in another direction.
- After the patient responds to the new resistance the therapist moves the other hand to resist the new direction.

Example: Trunk stability (Fig. 3.4 a):
▶ Combine traction with resistance to the patient's trunk flexor muscles. "Don't let me push you backward."
▶ When the patient is contracting his or her trunk flexor muscles, maintain the traction and resistance with one hand while moving your other hand to approximate and resist the patient's trunk extension. "Now don't let me pull you forward."
▶ As the patient responds to the new resistance, move the hand that was still resisting trunk flexion to resist trunk extension.
▶ Reverse directions as often as needed to be sure the patient is stable. "Now don't let me push you. Don't let me pull you."

Modifications

- The technique can begin with slow reversals and progress to smaller ranges until the patient is stabilizing.
- The stabilization can start with the stronger muscle groups to facilitate the weaker muscles.
- The resistance may be moved around the patient so that all muscle groups work (Fig. 3.4 b).

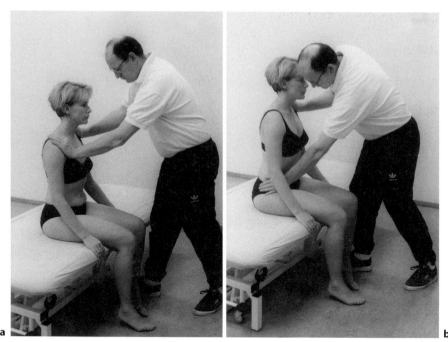

a   b

Fig. 3.4 a,b. Stabilizing Reversal for the trunk. **a** Stabilizing the upper trunk. **b** One hand continues resisting the upper trunk, the therapist's other hand changes to resist at the pelvis

Example: Trunk and neck stability:
▶ After the upper trunk is stable, you may give resistance at the pelvis to stabilize the lower trunk.
▶ Next you may move one hand to resist neck extension.

Note: The speed of the reversal may be increased or decreased.

→ Points to remember
  ● Starting working in the strongest direction
  ● You can begin with slow reversals and decrease the range until the patient is stabilizing

3.3.3 Rhythmic Stabilization

Characterization

Alternating isometric contractions against resistance, no motion intended.[2]

Goals

- Increase active and passive range of motion
- Increase strength
- Increase stability and balance
- Decrease pain

Indications and contraindications

Indications

- Limited range of motion
- Pain, particularly when motion is attempted
- Joint instability
- Weakness in the antagonistic muscle group
- Decreased balance

Contraindications

- Cerebellar involvement (Kabat 1950)
- The patient is unable to follow instructions due to age, language difficulty, cerebral dysfunction

Description

- The therapist resists an isometric contraction of the agonistic muscle group. The patient maintains the position of the part without trying to move.
- The resistance is increased slowly as the patient builds a matching force.
- When the patient is responding fully, the therapist moves one hand to begin resisting the antagonistic motion at the distal part. Neither the therapist nor the patient relaxes as the resistance changes (Fig. 3.5).
- The new resistance is built up slowly. As the patient responds the therapist moves the other hand to resist the antagonistic motion also.
- Use traction or approximation as indicated by the patient's condition.

---

[2] In the first and second editions of Proprioceptive neuromuscular facilitation, Knott and Voss describe this technique as resisting alternately the agonistic and antagonistic patterns without relaxation. In the third edition (1985), Voss et al. describe resisting the agonistic pattern distally and the antagonistic pattern proximally.

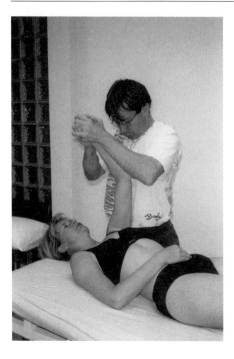

Fig. 3.5. Rhythmic Stabilization of the shoulder in the diagonal of flexion-abduction/extension-adduction

- The reversals are repeated as often as needed.
- Use a static command. "Stay there." "Don't try to move."

Example: Trunk stability:

▶ Resist an isometric contraction of the patient's trunk flexor muscles. "Stay still, match my resistance in front."

▶ Next, take all the anterior resistance with your left hand and move your right hand to resist trunk extension. "Now start matching me in back, hold it."

▶ As the patient responds to the new resistance, move your left hand to resist trunk extension. "Stay still, match me in back."

- The direction of contraction may be reversed as often as necessary to reach the chosen goal. "Now hold in front again. Stay still. Now start matching me in the back."

Modifications

- The technique can begin with the stronger group of muscles for facilitation of the weaker muscle group (successive induction).
- The stabilizing activity can be followed by a strengthening technique for the weak muscles.

- To increase the range of motion the stabilization may be followed by asking the patient to move farther into the restricted range.
- For relaxation the patient may be asked to relax all muscles at the end of the technique.
- To gain relaxation without pain the technique may be done with muscles distant from the painful area.

Example: Trunk stability and strengthening:

▶ Resist alternate trunk flexion and extension until the patient is stabile.
▶ When the trunk is stabile, give increased stabilizing resistance to the stronger direction ("Match me in back" for extension).
▶ Then ask for motion into the direction to be strengthened ("Now push me forward as hard as you can" to strengthen flexion).

Table 3.1

Differences between Stabilizing Reversals and Rhythmic Stabilization	
Stabilizing Reversals	**Rhythmic Stabilization**
Isotonic muscle action	Isometric muscle action
Intention to move	No intention to move
Dynamic command	Static command
Change from one part of the body to another part is allowed	Only one part of the body is treated
Muscle activity: Agonist to antagonist to agonist to antagonist	Muscle activity: Agonistic and antagonistic activity (possible co-contraction)

→ **Points to remember**
- Use static commands because no motion intended
- The stabilization may be done with muscles distant from a painful area
- Stabilization can be followed by a strengthening technique

3.4 Repeated Stretch (Repeated Contractions)

3.4.1 Repeated Stretch from Beginning of Range

Characterization

The stretch reflex elicited from muscles under the tension of elongation.

! Note: Only muscles should be under tension; take care not to stretch the joint structures.

Goals

- Facilitate initiation of motion
- Increase active range of motion
- Increase strength
- Prevent or reduce fatigue
- Guide motion in the desired direction

Indications and Contraindications

Indications

- Weakness
- Inability to initiate motion due to weakness or rigidity
- Fatigue
- Decreased awareness of motion

Contraindications

- Joint instability
- Pain
- Unstable bones due to fracture or osteoporosis
- Damaged muscle or tendon

Description

- Lengthened muscle tension = stretch stimulus
- Lengthened muscle tension + tap = stretch reflex
  - ▶ The therapist gives a preparatory command while fully elongating the muscles in the pattern. Pay particular attention to the rotation.
  - ▶ Give a quick "tap" to lengthen (stretch) the muscles further and evoke the stretch reflex.
  - ▶ At the same time as the stretch reflex, give a command to link the patient's voluntary effort to contract the stretched muscles with the reflex response.
  - ▶ Resist the resulting reflex and voluntary muscle contraction.

Example: Stretch of the pattern of flexion–abduction–internal rotation:
- ▶ Place the foot in plantar flexion–inversion then rotate the patient's lower extremity into external rotation and the hip into full extension, adduction, and external rotation.
- ▶ When all the muscles of the flexion–abduction–internal rotation pattern are taut, give the preparatory command "Now!" while quickly elongating (stretching) all the muscles farther.
- ▶ Immediately after the stretch, give the command "Pull up and out."

▶ When you feel the patient's muscles contract, give resistance to the entire pattern.

Modifications

- The technique may be repeated, without stopping, from the beginning of the range as soon as the contraction weakens or stops.
- The resistance may be modified so that only some motions are allowed to occur (timing for emphasis). For example, the therapist may prevent any hip motion from occurring while resisting the ankle dorsiflexion and eversion through its range.

> → **Points to remember**
> - **Combine the stretch reflex with the patient's voluntary effort**
> - **Wait for the resulting muscle contraction, then resist**

3.4.2 Repeated Stretch Through Range

Characterization

The stretch reflex elicited from muscles under the tension of contraction (Fig. 3.6).

Goals

- Increase active range of motion
- Increase strength
- Prevent or reduce fatigue
- Guide motion in the desired direction

Indications and Contraindications

Indications

- Weakness
- Fatigue
- Decreased awareness of desired motion

Contraindications

- Joint instability
- Pain
- Unstable bones due to fracture or osteoporosis
- Damaged muscle or tendon

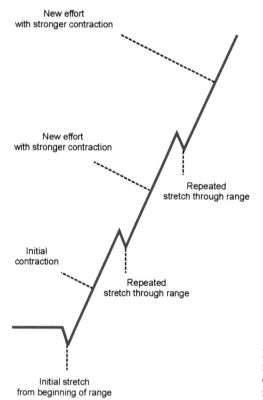

New effort
with stronger contraction

New effort
with stronger contraction

Repeated
stretch through range

Initial
contraction

Repeated
stretch through range

Initial stretch
from beginning of range

Fig. 3.6. Repeated Stretch through range: stretch reflex at the beginning of the range and repeated stretch reflex through range

Description

- The therapist resists a pattern of motion so all the muscles are contracting and tense. You can start with an initial stretch reflex.
- Next give a preparatory command to coordinate the stretch reflex with a new and increased effort by the patient.
- At the same time you slightly elongate (stretch) the muscles by momentarily giving too much resistance.
- A new and stronger muscle contraction is asked for and resisted.
- The stretch reflex is repeated to strengthen the contraction or redirect the motion as the patient moves through the range.
- The patient must be allowed to move before the next stretch reflex is given.
- The patient must not relax or reverse direction during the stretch.

Example: Repeated Stretch of the lower extremity pattern of flexion–abduction–internal rotation

▶ Resist the patient's moving his or her lower extremity into flexion–abduction–internal rotation. "Foot up, pull your leg up and out."

▶ Give a preparatory command ("Now!") while slightly over-resisting the motion so that you pull the patient's leg a short distance back in the direction of extension–adduction–external rotation. The patient must maintain the contraction of the stretched muscles.

▶ Give the command "Pull again, harder" immediately after the stretch.

▶ Give appropriate resistance to the increased contraction that follows the re-stretch of the muscles.

▶ Repeat the stretch and resistance if you feel the patient's strength decreasing.

▶ Repeat the stretch reflex if you feel the patient start to move in the wrong direction.

▶ Always allow a response to occur before giving another re-stretch. A rule of thumb is three to four re-stretches during one pattern.

Modifications

- The therapist may ask for a stabilizing contraction of the pattern before re-stretching the muscles. "Hold your leg here, don't let me pull it down. Now, pull it up harder."
- The therapist may resist a stabilizing contraction of the stronger muscles in the pattern while re-stretching and resisting the weaker muscles (timing for emphasis).

Example: Repeated contractions of ankle dorsiflexion and eversion with the hip motion stabilized.

▶ "Lock in" the hip motion by resisting a stabilizing contraction of those muscles. "Hold your hip there."

▶ The ankle motion of dorsiflexion and eversion is re-stretched and the new contraction resisted through range. "Pull your ankle up and out harder."

→ **Points to remember**
- **A new and stronger muscle contraction should follow each re-stretch**
- **The patient must be allowed to move before the next stretch reflex is given**
- **A rule of thumb is three to four re-stretches during one pattern**

3.5 Contract-Relax

We refer to the resisting patterns or muscles as "antagonists", and the opposite patterns or muscles as "agonists".

3.5.1 Contract-Relax: Direct Treatment

Characterization

Resisted isotonic contraction of the restricting muscles (antagonists) followed by relaxation and movement into the increased range.

Goal

• Increased passive range of motion

Indication

• Decreased passive range of motion

Description

• The therapist or the patient moves the joint or body segment to the end of the passive range of motion. Active motion or motion against a little resistance is preferred.
• The therapist asks the patient for a strong contraction of the restricting muscle or pattern (antagonists). (The authors feel that the contraction should be held for at least 5–8 seconds) (Fig. 3.7 a)
• Enough motion is allowed for the therapist to be certain that all the desired muscles, particularly the rotators, are contracting.
• After sufficient time, the therapist tells the patient to relax.
• Both the patient and the therapist relax.
• The joint or body part is repositioned, either actively by the patient or passively by the therapist, to the new limit of the passive range. Active motion is preferred and may be resisted.
• The technique is repeated until no more range is gained.
• Active resisted exercise of the agonistic and antagonistic muscles in the new range of motion finishes the activity.

Example: Increasing the range of shoulder flexion, abduction, and external rotation.
• The patient moves the arm to the end of the range of flexion–abduction–external rotation. "Open your hand and lift your arm up as high as you can."
• Resist an isotonic contraction of the pattern of extension–adduction–internal rotation. "Squeeze my hand and pull your arm down and across. Keep turning your hand down."

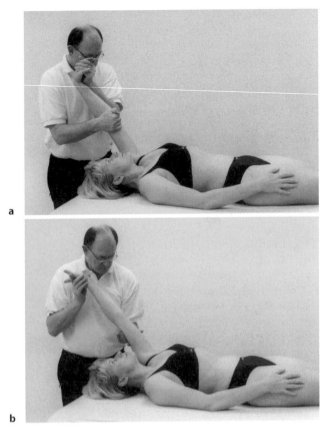

Fig. 3.7 a, b. Hold-Relax or Contract-Relax. **a** Direct treatment for shortened shoulder extensor and adductor muscles. **b** Indirect treatment for shortened shoulder extensor and adductor muscles

- Allow enough motion to occur for both you and the patient to know that all the muscles in the pattern, particularly the rotators, are contracting. "Keep pulling your arm down."
- After resisting the contraction (for a sufficient amount of time), both you and the patient relax. "Relax, let everything go loose."
- Now, resist the patient's motion into the newly gained range. "Open your hand and lift your arm up farther."
- When no more range is gained, exercise the agonistic and antagonistic patterns, either in the new range or throughout the entire range of motion. "Squeeze and pull your arm down; now open your hand and lift your arm up again."

Modifications

- The patient is asked to move immediately into the desired range without any relaxation.
- Alternating contractions (reversals) of agonistic and antagonistic muscles may be done. "Keep your arm still, don't let me pull it up. Now don't let me push your arm down."

3.5.2 Contract-Relax: Indirect Treatment

Description

- The technique uses contraction of the agonistic muscles instead of the shortened muscles. "Don't let me push your arm down, keep pushing up." (Fig. 3.7 b).

Indication

- Use the indirect method when the contraction of the restricting muscles is too painful or too weak to produce an effective contraction.

→ **Points to remember**
- **The technique is only to increase passive range of motion**
- **The patient's active motion is always preferred**
- **When the contraction of the restricting (antagonist) muscles is painful or weak, use the agonist**

3.6 Hold-Relax

We refer to the resisting patterns or muscles as "antagonists", and the opposite patterns or muscles as "agonists".

3.6.1 Hold-Relax: Direct Treatment

Characterization

Resisted isometric contraction of the antagonistic muscles (shortened muscles) followed by relaxation (Fig. 3.7 a).

Goals

- Increase passive range of motion
- Decrease pain

Indications and Contraindication

Indications

- Decreased passive range of motion
- Pain
- The patient's isotonic contractions are too strong for the therapist to control

Contraindication

- The patient is unable to do an isometric contraction

Description

For increasing range of motion
- The therapist or patient moves the joint or body segment to the end of the passive or pain-free range of motion. Active motion is preferred. The therapist may resist if that does not cause pain.

! **Note: If this position is very painful the patient should move slightly out of position until it is no longer painful.**

- The therapist asks for an isometric contraction of the restricting muscle or pattern (antagonists) with emphasis on rotation. (The authors feel that the contraction should be maintained for at least 5–8 seconds)
- The resistance is increased slowly.
- No motion is intended by either the patient or the therapist.
- After holding the contraction for enough time the therapist asks the patient to relax.
- Both the therapist and the patient relax gradually.
- The joint or body part is repositioned either actively or passively to the new limit of range. Active motion is preferred if it is pain-free. The motion may be resisted if that does not cause pain.
- Repeat all steps in the new limit of range.

Description

- For decreasing pain
- The patient is in a position of comfort
- The therapist resists an isometric contraction of muscles affecting the painful segment

→ **Points to remember**
- **The patient's active motion is always preferred**
- **Both the therapist and the patient must relax**

3.6.2 Hold-Relax: Indirect Treatment

In the indirect treatment with Hold-Relax you resist the synergists of the shortened or painful muscles and not the painful muscles or painful motion. If that still causes pain, resist the synergistic muscles *of the opposite pattern* instead (Fig. 3.7b).

Indication

• When the contraction of the restricted muscles is too painful.

Description

• The patient is in a position of comfort.
• The therapist resists isometric contractions of *synergistic* muscles distant from the painful segment.
• The resistance is built up slowly and remains at a level below that which causes pain.
• During relaxation the resistance decreases slowly.

Example: Indirect treatment for decreasing pain in the right shoulder and relaxation of the shoulder internal rotator muscles.
▶ The patient lies with his or her right arm supported in a comfortable position and the right elbow flexed.
▶ Hold the patient's right hand and ask for an isometric contraction of the ulnar flexor muscles of the wrist. "Keep your hand and wrist right there. Match my resistance."
▶ Resist an isometric contraction of the ulnar wrist flexor muscles and forearm pronator muscles. Build the resistance up slowly and keep it at a pain-free level. "Keep holding, match my resistance."
▶ While maintaining the resistance, monitor muscle activity in the patient's right shoulder, particularly the internal rotation.
▶ Both you and the patient relax slowly and completely. "Now let go slowly all over."
▶ Both you and the patient breathe
▶ Repeat the technique in the same position to gain more relaxation, or move the forearm into more supination or pronation to change the effect on the shoulder muscles.

Modifications

• The technique may be done with contraction of the synergistic muscles *of the opposite pattern,* in this case resisting an isometric contraction of the radial extensor muscles of the wrist and the forearm supinator muscles.
• Alternating isometric contractions or Rhythmic Stabilization may be done.

- If the patient is unable to do an isometric contraction, carefully controlled stabilizing contractions may be used. The therapist's resistance and the patient's effort must stay at a level that does not cause pain.

> → **Points to remember**
>   - **Resist the synergists of the shortened or painful muscle**
>   - **Both therapist and patient keep breathing**
>   - **The effort stays at a level that does not cause pain**

3.7 Replication

Characterization

A technique to facilitate motor learning of functional activities. Teaching the patient the outcome of a movement or activity is important for functional work (for example sports) and self-care activities.

Goals

- Teach the patient the end position (outcome) of the movement.
- Assess the patient's ability to sustain a contraction when the agonist muscles are shortened.

Description

- Place the patient in the "end" position of the activity where all the agonist muscles are shortened.
- The patient holds that position while the therapist resists all the components. Use all the basic procedures to facilitate the patient's muscles.
- Ask the patient to relax. Move the patient, passively a short distance back in the opposite direction, then ask the patient to return to the 'end' position.
- For each replication of the movement start farther toward the beginning of the movement to challenge the patient through a greater range of the motion.

> → **Points to remember**
>   - **Exercise or teach functional activities**
>   - **Use all the Basic Procedures for facilitation**

3.8 PNF Techniques and Their Goals

Suggestions for PNF techniques that can be used to achieve a particular goal are outlined below.

1. Initiate motion
   ▶ Rhythmic Initiation
   ▶ Repeated Stretch from beginning of range
2. Learn a motion
   ▶ Rhythmic Initiation
   ▶ Combination of Isotonics
   ▶ Repeated Stretch from beginning of range
   ▶ Repeated Stretch through range
   ▶ Replication
3. Change rate of motion
   ▶ Rhythmic Initiation
   ▶ Dynamic Reversals
   ▶ Repeated Stretch from beginning of range
   ▶ Repeated Stretch through range
4. Increase strength
   ▶ Combination of Isotonics
   ▶ Dynamic Reversals
   ▶ Rhythmic Stabilization
   ▶ Stabilizing Reversals
   ▶ Repeated Stretch from beginning of range
   ▶ Repeated Stretch through range
5. Increase stability
   ▶ Combination of Isotonics
   ▶ Stabilizing Reversals
   ▶ Rhythmic Stabilization
6. Increase coordination and control
   ▶ Combination of Isotonics
   ▶ Rhythmic Initiation
   ▶ Dynamic Reversals
   ▶ Stabilizing Reversals
   ▶ Rhythmic Stabilization
   ▶ Repeated Stretch from beginning of range
   ▶ Replication
7. Increase endurance
   ▶ Dynamic Reversals
   ▶ Stabilizing Reversals
   ▶ Rhythmic Stabilization
   ▶ Repeated Stretch from beginning of range
   ▶ Repeated Stretch through range

8. Increase range of motion
   ▸ Dynamic Reversals
   ▸ Stabilizing Reversals
   ▸ Rhythmic Stabilization
   ▸ Repeated Stretch from beginning of range
   ▸ Contract-Relax
   ▸ Hold-Relax
9. Relaxation
   ▸ Rhythmic Initiation
   ▸ Rhythmic Stabilization
   ▸ Hold-Relax
10. Decrease pain
   ▸ Rhythmic Stabilization (or Stabilizing Reversals)
   ▸ Hold-Relax

References

Kabat H (1950) Studies on neuromuscular dysfunction, XII: Rhythmic stabilization; a new and more effective technique for treatment of paralysis through a cerebellar mechanism. Perm Found Med Bull 8: 9–19

Knott M, Voss DE (1956) Proprioceptive neuromuscular facilitation: patterns and techniques. Harper and Row, New York

Knott M, Voss DE (1968) Proprioceptive neuromuscular facilitation: patterns and techniques. 2nd edn. Harper and Row, New York

Sullivan PE, Markos PD, Minor MAD (1982) An integrated approach to therapeutic exercise. Reston, Virginia

Voss DE, Ionta M, Myer BT (1985) Proprioceptive neuromuscular facilitation, patterns and techniques. 3rd edn. Harper and Row, New York

Further Reading

Markos PD (1979) Ipsilateral and contralateral effects of proprioceptive neuromuscular facilitation techniques on hip motion and electro-myographic activity. Phys Ther 59 (11): 1366–1373

Moore M, Kukulkan C (1988) Depression of H reflexes following voluntary contraction. Phys Ther 68:862

Rose-Jacobs R, Gilberti N (1984) Effect of PNF and Rood relaxation techniques on muscle length. Phys Ther 64:725

Sady SP, Wortman M, Blanke D (1982) Flexibility training: ballistic, static or proprioceptive neuromuscular facilitation? Arch Phys Med Rehabil 63:261–263

Tanigawa MC (1972) Comparison of the hold-relax procedure and passive mobilization on increasing muscle length. Phys Ther 52:725–735

4 Patient Treatment

Planning treatment is a *systematic process* to develop the most appropriate treatment for each patient (Sullivan et al. 1982). Our treatment seeks to help each patient gain the highest level of function possible.

❑ **Definition.** The PNF philosophy means we mobilize the patient's reserves through a positive approach toward the total human being during intensive functional training.

An effective treatment depends on our doing a complete and accurate *evaluation* to identify the patient's areas of function and dysfunction. Based on this evaluation we set general and specific *goals*, both immediate and for the long term. We also ascertain the patient's personal goals. Then we design a *treatment plan* to achieve those goals. *Continuous assessment* guides us in adjusting the treatment as the patient progresses.

4.1 Evaluation

Working within the PNF philosophy, we look first for the patient's areas of function. We will use this knowledge of the patient's abilities, strong areas and the patient's own goals to construct effective treatments.

Next we note the patient's general (functional) problems. Last, we identify the specific dysfunctions that are causing the general problems.
- Areas of function
  a. Pain free
  b. Strong
  c. Able to move and stabilize
  d. Motion is controlled and coordinated
- Dysfunctions
  a. General (functional) loss
    ▶ Static: loss of the ability to maintain a position
    ▶ Dynamic: loss of the ability to move or control motion

b. Specific deficits (the reasons for the functional losses)
- ▶ Pain
- ▶ Decreased range of motion due to:
  1. joint restrictions
  2. muscle tightness or contracture
- ▶ Weakness
- ▶ Loss of sensation or proprioception
- ▶ Deficits in sight, hearing
- ▶ Deficient motor control
- ▶ Lack of endurance

4.2 Treatment Goals

After doing the evaluation, we set both the general and the specific treatment goals.

❑ General goals are expressed as functional activities. These goals are not limits, we change them as the patient improves.

❑ Specific goals are set for each treatment activity and for each treatment session.

Examples of general goals and one specific treatment goal for each patient example.

1. Static dysfunction: A patient who has difficulty maintaining standing balance after suffering a head injury.
   - ▶ General goal: The patient can stand without support while doing functional upper extremity activities.
   - ▶ Specific treatment goal: The patient can maintain a steady bridging position without using the arms for 30 seconds. (Begin treatment in a more stable and less threatening position.)
2. Dynamic dysfunction due to pain: A patient who has pain in his right knee after miniscus injury.
   - ▶ General goal: The patient will be able to run one mile (1.6 km) in less than 6 minutes without pain in the knee.
   - ▶ Specific treatment goal: The patient can hold a one-leg bridging position on the right leg with the left leg extended for 30 seconds. (Begin treatment with limited weight-bearing on the right leg.)
3. Dynamic dysfunction due to the loss of ability to move: A patient who has had a stroke with resultant hemiplegia.
   - ▶ General goal: The patient will be able to walk 25 feet (8 m) in 2 minutes using a cane and an ankle-foot orthosis.
   - ▶ Specific treatment goal: The patient can shift weight from the right to the left ischial tuberosity while sitting without any support. (Begin treatment with weight shifting in a stable position.)

4.3 Treatment Planning and Treatment Design

PNF uses muscle contractions to affect the body. If muscle contractions are not appropriate for the patient's condition or if their use does not achieve the desired goals, the therapist should use other methods. Modalities such as heat and cold, passive joint motion, and soft tissue mobilization may be combined with PNF for effective treatment.

Selection of the most effective treatment depends on the condition of the patient's muscles and joints and any existing medical problems. The therapist combines and modifies the procedures and the techniques to suit the needs of each patient. Treatment should be intensive, mobilizing the patient's reserves without resulting in pain or fatigue.

4.3.1 Specific Patient Needs

The therapist lists the patient's needs. For example:
1. Decrease pain
2. Increase range of motion
3. Increase strength, coordination, and control of motion
4. Develop a proper balance between motion and stability
5. Increase endurance

4.3.2 Designing the Treatment

The therapist designs a treatment to meet the patient's needs. Factors to be considered include:
1. Direct or indirect treatment
2. Appropriate activities
   ▶ Movement or stability
   ▶ What types of muscle contractions
3. The best position for the patient. Consider:
   ▶ The patient's comfort and security
   ▶ The effect of gravity
   ▶ The effect on two-joint muscles
   ▶ Progression of treatment
   ▶ Reflex facilitation
   ▶ Use of vision
   ▶ Closed chain or open chain muscle work
   ▶ Position to decrease spasticity
4. Techniques and procedures
5. Patterns and combinations of patterns
6. Functional and goal oriented tasks

4.4 Assessment

The process of patient evaluation and the assessment of treatment is continuous. By assessing the results after each treatment, the therapist can determine the effectiveness of both that treatment activity and treatment session and can then modify the treatment as necessary to achieve the stated goals.

Treatment modifications may include:
1. Changing the treatment procedures or the techniques
2. Increasing or decreasing facilitation by changing the use of:
    ▶ Reflexes
    ▶ Manual contact
    ▶ Visual cues
    ▶ Verbal cues
    ▶ Traction and approximation
3. Increasing or decreasing the resistance given
4. Working with the patient in positions of function
5. Progressing to more complex activities

4.5 Direct and Indirect Treatment

4.5.1 Direct Treatment

Direct treatment may involve:
1. Use of treatment techniques on the affected limb, muscle, or motion.

Example: To gain increased range in the shoulder motions of flexion, abduction, and external rotation, the therapist treats the involved shoulder using the technique Contract-Relax on the tight pectoralis major muscle.

2. Directing the patient's attention to stabilizing or moving the affected segment.

Example: While the patient stands on the involved leg, the therapist gives approximation through the pelvis to facilitate weight-bearing.

4.5.2 Indirect Treatment

Many studies have shown the effectiveness of indirect treatment that begins on *strong and pain-free parts* of the body. Hellebrandt et al. (1947) reported the development of muscle tension in unexercised parts of the body during and after maximal exercise of one limb. Other experiments have described electromyographic (EMG) activity in the agonistic and antagonistic muscles of the contralateral upper or lower extremity during resisted isotonic and isometric exercise (Moore 1975; Devine et al. 1981; Pink 1981). The trunk musculature can also be exercised indirectly. For example, the abdominal muscles contract synergistically when a person raises his arm. This activity occurs in normal subjects and in patients suffering from central nervous system disorders as well (Angel and Eppler 1967). An increased passive range of motion can be gained indirectly by using Contract-Relax on uninvolved areas of the body (Markos 1979).

To give the patient maximum benefit from indirect treatment the therapist resists strong movements or patterns. Maximum strengthening occurs when the patient's strong limbs work in combination with the weak ones. When pain is a presenting symptom, treatment focuses on pain-free areas of the body. Using carefully guided and controlled irradiation the therapist can treat the affected limb or joint without risk of increasing the pain or injury.

Indirect treatment may involve:
- Use of the techniques on an unaffected or less affected part of the body. The therapist directs the irradiation into the affected area to achieve the desired results.

Example: To gain range in shoulder flexion, abduction and external rotation.
▶ The therapist resists an isometric contraction of the ulnar wrist flexor and the pronator muscles of the affected arm.
▶ After resisting the contraction, the therapist and the patient relax.
▶ This use of Hold Relax will produce a contraction and relaxation of the ipsilateral pectoralis major muscle. The treated arm need not be moved but may remain in a position of comfort.

- Directing the patient's attention and effort toward working with the less affected parts of the body.

Example: To improve lower extremity weight bearing.
▶ While the patient sits with both feet on the floor, the therapist resists the "lifting" pattern (trunk extension) on the side of the involved lower extremity.
▶ This produces contraction of the extensor muscles in the lower extremities and increased weight-bearing through the ipsilateral ischial tuberosity and the foot.

4.6 Treatment Examples

The following examples of procedures, techniques, and combinations to treat specific patient problems should not be interpreted as definitive but only as guidelines. Let your imagination and the patient's condition be your guides.
1. Pain
   a) Procedures
      ▶ Indirect treatment
      ▶ Resistance below that which produces pain or stress
      ▶ Isometric muscle contraction
      ▶ Bilateral work
      ▶ Traction
      ▶ Position for comfort

b) Techniques
- ▶ Rhythmic Stabilization
- ▶ Hold-Relax
- ▶ Stabilizing Reversals

c) Combinations
- ▶ Hold-Relax followed by Combination of Isotonics
- ▶ Rhythmic Stabilization followed by Slow Reversal (Dynamic Reversals) moving first toward the painful range

2. Decreased strength and active range of motion
   a) Procedures
   - ▶ Appropriate resistance
   - ▶ Timing for emphasis
   - ▶ Stretch
   - ▶ Traction or approximation
   - ▶ Patient position

   b) Techniques
   - ▶ Repeated Stretch from beginning of range
   - ▶ Repeated Stretch through range (Repeated Contractions)
   - ▶ Combination of Isotonics
   - ▶ Dynamic (slow) Reversal of Antagonists
     1. Facilitation from stronger antagonists
     2. Prevention and relief of fatigue

   c) Combinations
   - ▶ Dynamic Reversal of Antagonists combined with Repeated Stretch through range (Repeated Contractions) of the weak pattern
   - ▶ Rhythmic Stabilization at a strong point in the range of motion followed by Repeated Contractions of the weak pattern

3. Decreased passive range of motion
   a) Procedures
   - ▶ Timing for emphasis
   - ▶ Traction
   - ▶ Appropriate resistance

   b) Techniques
   - ▶ Contract-Relax or Hold-Relax
   - ▶ Stabilizing Reversal of Antagonists
   - ▶ Rhythmic Stabilization

   c) Combinations
   - ▶ Contract-Relax followed by Combination of Isotonics in the new range
   - ▶ Contract-Relax followed by Slow Reversals, beginning with motion into the new range
   - ▶ Rhythmic Stabilization or Stabilizing Reversals followed by Dynamic Reversal of Antagonists

4. Coordination and control
   a) Procedures
   - ▶ Patterns of facilitation

▶ Manual contact (grip)
▶ Vision
▶ Proper verbal cues, decreased cueing as patient progresses
▶ Decreasing facilitation as the patient progresses
b) Techniques
  ▶ Rhythmic Initiation
  ▶ Combination of Isotonics
  ▶ Dynamic Reversal of Antagonists
  ▶ Stabilizing Reversals
  ▶ Replication
c) Combinations
  ▶ Rhythmic Initiation, progressing to Combination of Isotonics
  ▶ Rhythmic Initiation done as reversals, progressing to Reversal of Antagonists
  ▶ Combination of Isotonics combined with Stabilizing or Dynamic Reversal of Antagonists

5. Stability and balance
a) Procedures
  ▶ Approximation
  ▶ Vision
  ▶ Manual contact (grip)
  ▶ Appropriate verbal commands
b) Techniques
  ▶ Stabilizing Reversals
  ▶ Combination of Isotonics
  ▶ Rhythmic Stabilization
c) Combinations
  ▶ Dynamic Reversal of Antagonists progressing to Stabilizing Reversals
  ▶ Dynamic Reversals (eccentric) progressing to Stabilizing Reversals

6. Endurance
Increasing the patient's general endurance is a part of all treatments. Varying the activity or exercise being done and changing the activity to a different muscle group or part of the body will enable the patient to work longer and harder. Attention to breathing while exercising as well as specific breathing exercises work to increase endurance.
a) Procedure
  ▶ Stretch reflex
b) Technique
  ▶ Reversal of antagonists
  ▶ Repeated Stretch and Repeated Contractions

References

Angel RW, Eppler WG Jr (1967) Synergy of contralateral muscles in normal subjects and patients with neurologic disease. Arch Phys Med Rehabil 48:233–239

Devine KL, LeVeau BF, Yack J (1981) Electromyographic activity recorded from an unexercised muscle during maximal isometric exercise of the contralateral agonists and antagonist. Phys Ther 61:898–903

Hellebrandt FA, Parrish AM, Houtz SJ (1947) Cross education, the influence of unilateral exercise on the contralateral limb. Arch Phys Med Rehabil 28:76–85

Markos PD (1979) Ipsilateral and contralateral effects of proprioceptive neuromuscular facilitation techniques on hip motion and electromyographic activity. Phys Ther 59(11): 1366–1373

Moore JC (1975) Excitation overflow: an electromyographic investigation. Arch Phys Med Rehabil 59:115–120

Pink M (1981) Contralateral effects of upper extremity proprioceptive neuromuscular facilitation patterns. Phys Ther 61(8):1158–1162

Sullivan PE, Markos PD, Minor MAD (1982) An integrated approach to therapeutic exercise, theory and clinical application. Reston Publishing Company, Reston VA

Further Reading

Exercise

Engle RP, Canner GG (1989) Proprioceptive neuromuscular facilitation (PNF) and modified procedures for anterior cruciate ligament (ACL) instability. J Orthop Sports Phys Ther 11:230–236

Hellebrandt FA (1951) Cross education: ipsilateral and contralateral effects of unimanual training. J Appl Physiol 4:135–144

Hellebrandt FA, Hautz SJ (1950) Influence of bimanual exercise on unilateral work capacity. J Appl Physiol 2:446–452

Hellebrandt FA Houtz SJ (1958) Methods of muscle training: the influence of pacing. Phys Ther 38:319–322

Hellebrandt FA, Houtz SJ, Eubank RN (1951) Influence of alternate and reciprocal exercise on work capacity. Arch Phys Med Rehabil 32:766–776

Hellebrandt FA, Houtz SJ, Hockman DE, Partridge MJ (1956) Physiological effects of simultaneous static and dynamic exercise. Am J Phys Med Rehabil 35:106–117

Nelson AG, Chambers RS, McGown CM, Penrose KW (1986) Proprioceptive neuromuscular facilitation versus weight training for enhancement of muscular strength and athletic performance. J Orthop Sports Phys Ther 8:250–253

Osternig LR, Robertson RN, Troxel RK, Hansen P (1990) Differential responses to proprioceptive neuromuscular facilitation (PNF) stretch techniques. Med Sci Sports Exerc 22: 106–111

Partridge MJ (1962) Repetitive resistance exercise: a method of indirect muscle training. Phys Ther 42:233–239

Pink M (1981) Contralateral effects of upper extremity proprioceptive neuromuscular facilitation patterns. Phys Ther 61:1158–1162

Richardson C, Toppenberg R, Jull G (1990) An initial evaluation of eight abdominal exercises for their ability to provide stabilization for the lumbar spine. Aust Physiother 36: 6–11

Hemiplegia

Brodal A (1973) Self–observations and neuro–anatomical considerations after a stroke. Brain 96:675–694

Duncan PW, Nelson SG (1983) Weakness – a primary motor deficit in hemiplegia. Neurol Rep 7 (1):3–4

Harro CC (1985) Implications of motor unit characteristics to speed of movement in hemiplegia. Neurol Rep 9 (3):55–61

Tang A, Rymer WZ (1981) Abnormal force – EMG relations in paretic limbs of hemiparetic human subjects. J Neurol Neurosurg Psychiatry 44:690–698

Trueblood PR, Walker JM, Perry J, Gronley JK (1988) Pelvic exercise and gait in hemiplegia. Phys Ther 69:32–40

Whitley DA, Sahrmann SA, Norton BJ (1982) Patterns of muscle activity in the hemiplegic upper extremity. Phys Ther 62:641

Winstein CJ, Jewell MJ, Montgomery J, Perry J, Thomas L (1982) Short leg casts: an adjunct to gait training hemiplegics. Phys Ther 64:713–714

Motor Control and Motor Learning

APTA (1991) Movement science: an American Physical Therapy Association monograph. APTA, Alexandria VA

APTA (1991) Contemporary management of motor control problems. Proceedings of the II Step conference. Foundation for Physical Therapy, Alexandria VA

Hellebrandt FA (1958) Application of the overload principle to muscle training in man. Arch Phys Med Rehabil 37:278–283

Light KE (1990) Information processing for motor performance in aging adults. Phys Ther 70 (12): 820–826

VanSant AF (1988) Rising from a supine position to erect stance: description of adult movement and a developmental hypothesis. Phys Ther 68 (2):185–192

VanSant AF (1990) Life-span development in functional tasks. Phys Ther 70 (12):788–798

Spasticity

Landau WM (1974) Spasticity: the fable of a neurological demon and the emperor's new therapy. Arch Neurol 31:217–219

Levine MG, Kabat H, Knott M, Voss DE (1954) Relaxation of spasticity by physiological techniques. Arch Phys Med Rehabil 35:214–223

Perry J (1980) Rehabilitation of spasticity. In: Felman RG, Young JRR, Koella WP (eds) Spasticity: disordered motor control. Year Book, Chicago

Sahrmann SA, Norton BJ (1977) The relationship of voluntary movement to spasticity in the upper motor neuron syndrome. Ann Neurol 2:460–465

Young RR, Wiegner AW (1987) Spasticity. Clin Orthop 219:50–62

Cold

Baker RJ, Bell GW (1991) The effect of therapeutic modalities on blood flow in the human
    calf. J Orthop Sports Phys Ther 13:23–27
Miglietta O (1964) Electromyographic characteristics of clonus and influence of cold. Arch
    Phys Med Rehabil 45:508–512
Miglietta O (1962) Evaluation of cold in spasticity. Am J Phys Med Rehabil 41:148–151
Olson JE, Stravino VD (1972) A review of cryotherapy. Phys Ther 52:840–853
Prentice WE Jr (1982) An electromyographic analysis of the effectiveness of heat or cold and
    stretching for inducing relaxation in injured muscle. J Orthop Sports Phys Ther 3: 133–140
Sabbahi MA, Powers WR (1981) Topical anesthesia: a possible treatment method for spasti-
    city. Arch Phys Med Rehabil 62:310–314

5 Patterns of Facilitation

Normal functional motion is composed of mass movement patterns of the limbs and the synergistic trunk muscles (Kabat 1960) (Fig. 5.1). The motor cortex generates and organizes these movement patterns, and the individual cannot voluntarily leave a muscle out of the movement pattern to which it belongs. This does not mean that we cannot contract muscles individually, but our discrete motions spring from the mass patterns (Beevor 1978; Kabat 1950). These *synergistic muscle combinations* form the PNF patterns of facilitation.

Some people believe that you must know and use the PNF patterns to work within the concept of PNF. We think that you need only the PNF philosophy

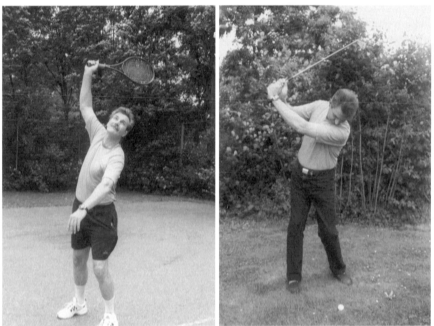

a   b

Fig. 5.1 a, b. Diagonal motions in sport: a tennis; b golf

and the appropriate procedures. The patterns, while not essential, are however valuable tools to have. Working with the synergistic relationships in the patterns allows problems to be treated indirectly. Also, the *stretch reflex* is more effective when an entire pattern rather than just the individual muscle is stretched.

The PNF patterns combine motion in all *three planes*:
1. The sagittal plane: flexion and extension
2. The coronal or frontal plane: abduction and adduction of limbs or lateral flexion of the spine
3. The transverse plane: rotation

We thus have motion that is "*spiral and diagonal*" (Knott and Voss 1968). Stretch and resistance reinforce the effectiveness of the patterns, as shown by an increased activity in the muscles. The increased muscular activity spreads both distally and proximally within a pattern and from one pattern to related patterns of motion (irradiation). Treatment uses irradiation from those synergistic combinations of muscles (patterns) to strengthen the desired muscle groups or reinforce the desired functional motions.

When we exercise in the patterns against resistance, all the muscles that are a part of the synergy will contract if they can. The rotational component of the pattern is the key to effective resistance. Correct resistance to rotation will strengthen the entire pattern. Too much resistance to rotation will prevent motion from occurring or "break" a stabilizing contraction.

The motion occurring at the proximal joint names the *patterns*, as in flexion-adduction-external rotation of the shoulder. Two antagonistic patterns make up a diagonal. For example, an upper extremity diagonal contains shoulder flexion-adduction-external rotation and the antagonist pattern extension-abduction-internal rotation. The proximal and distal joints of the limb are linked in the pattern. The middle joint is free to flex, extend or maintain its position. For example, finger flexion, radial flexion of the

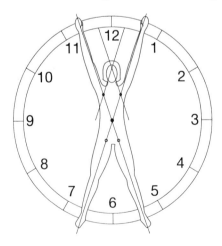

Fig. 5.2. Patterns are "spiral and diagonal" [modified from Klein-Vogelbach S (1990) Functional kinetics. Springer, Berlin Heidelberg New York]

wrist, and forearm supination are integral parts of the pattern of shoulder flexion-adduction-external rotation. The elbow, however, may flex, extend or remain in one position.

The trunk and limbs work together to form complete synergies. For example, the pattern of shoulder flexion-adduction-external rotation with anterior elevation of the scapula combines with trunk extension and rotation to the opposite side to complete a total motion. If you know the synergistic muscle combinations, you can work out the patterns. If you know the pattern, you will know the synergistic muscles. When an extremity is in its fully lengthened position the synergistic trunk muscles are also under tension. The therapist should feel tension in both the limb and trunk muscles.

The *groove* of the pattern is that line drawn by the hand or foot (distal component) as the limb moves through its range. For the head and neck, the groove is drawn by a plane through the nose, chin, and crown of the head. The groove for the upper trunk is drawn by the tip of the shoulder and for the lower trunk by the hip bone. Because the trunk and limbs work together, their grooves join or are parallel (Fig. 5.2). As discussed earlier, the therapist's body should be in line with or parallel to the relevant groove. Pictures of the complete patterns with the therapist in the proper position come in the following chapters.

To move concentrically through the entire range of a pattern:
- The limb is positioned in the "*lengthened range.*"
  - ▶ All the associated muscles (agonists) are lengthened.
  - ▶ There is no pain, and no joint stress.
  - ▶ The trunk does not rotate or roll.
- The limb moves into the "shortened range."
  - ▶ The end of the range of contraction of the muscles (agonists) is reached.
  - ▶ The antagonistic muscle groups are lengthened.
  - ▶ There is no pain and no joint stress.
  - ▶ The trunk did not rotate or roll.

The *normal timing* of an extremity pattern is:
- The distal part (hand and wrist or foot and ankle) moves through its full range first and holds its position.
- The other components move smoothly together so that they complete their movement almost simultaneously.
- Rotation is an integral part of the motion and is resisted from the beginning to the end of the motion.

We can vary the pattern in several ways:
- By changing the activity of the middle joint in the extremity pattern for function
  Example: First, the pattern of shoulder flexion-abduction-external rotation is done with the elbow moving from extension to flexion. The patient's

hand rubs his or her head. The next time, the same pattern is done with the elbow moving from a flexed to an extended position, so the patient's hand can reach for a high object.

- By changing the activity of the middle joint in the extremity pattern for the effect on two-joint muscles.
  Example: First, the pattern of hip flexion-adduction-external rotation is done with the knee moving from the extended to the flexed position. In this combination, the hamstring muscles shorten actively. Next time, the same pattern is used with the knee staying straight. This combination stretches the hamstring muscles.
- By changing the patient's position to change the effects of gravity.
  Example: The pattern of hip extension-abduction-internal rotation is done in a side lying position so the abductor muscles work against gravity.
- By changing the patient's position to a more functional one.
  Example: The upper extremity patterns are exercised in a sitting position and incorporate functional activities such as eating or combing the hair.
- By changing the patient's position to use visual cues.
  Example: Have the patient in a half-sitting position so that he or she can see the foot and ankle when exercising it.

We can combine the patterns in many ways. The emphasis of treatment is on the arms or legs when the limbs move independently. The emphasis is on the trunk when the arms are joined by one hand gripping the other arm or when the legs are touching and move together. Choosing how to combine the patterns for the greatest functional effect is a part of the assessment[1] and treatment planning.

We name the pattern combinations according to how the limb movements (arms, legs or both) relate to each other:

- *Unilateral*: one arm or one leg
- *Bilateral*: both arms, both legs, or combinations of arms and legs (Fig. 5.3):
  - ▶ *Symmetrical*: the limbs move in the same pattern (e.g., both move in flexion-abduction) (Fig. 5.3 a)
  - ▶ *Asymmetrical*: the limbs move in opposite patterns (e.g., the right limb moves in flexion-abduction, the left moves in flexion-adduction) (Fig. 5.3 b)
  - ▶ *Symmetrical reciprocal*: the limbs move in the same diagonal but opposite directions (e.g., the right limb moves in flexion-abduction, the left in extension-adduction) (Fig. 5.3 c)
  - ▶ *Asymmetrical reciprocal*: the limbs move in opposite diagonals and opposite directions (e.g., the right limb moves in flexion-abduction, the left in extension-abduction) (Fig. 5.3 d)

---

[1] To evaluate: to identify the patient's areas of function and dysfunction. To assess: to measure or judge the result of a treatment procedure.

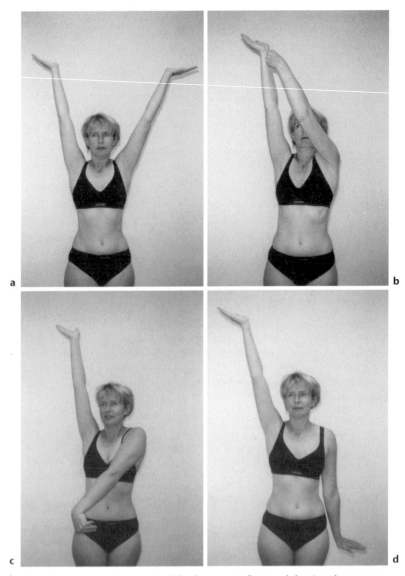

Fig. 5.3 a–d. Bilateral patterns. **a** Symmetrical: both arms in flexion-abduction. **b** Asymmetrical: right arm in flexion-abduction and left arm in flexion-adduction. **c** Symmetrical reciprocal: right arm in flexion-abduction and left arm in extension-adduction. **d** Asymmetrical reciprocal: right arm in flexion-abduction and left arm in extension-abduction

References

Beevor CE (1978) The Croonian lectures on muscular movements and their representation in the central nervous system. In: Payton OD, Hirt S, Newton RA (eds) Scientific basis for neurophysiologic approaches to therapeutic exercise: an anthology. Davis, Philadelphia

Kabat H (1950) Studies on neuromuscular dysfunction, XIII: new concepts and techniques of neuromuscular reeducation for paralysis. Perm Found Med Bull 8(3):121–143

Kabat H (1960) Central mechanisms for recovery of neuromuscular function. Science 112: 23–24

Knott M, Voss DE (1968) Proprioceptive neuromuscular facilitation: patterns and techniques, 2nd edn. Harper and Row, New York

Further Reading

Bosma JF, Gellhorn E (1946) Electromyographic studies of muscular co-ordination on stimulation of motor cortex. J Neurophysiol 9:263–274

Gellhorn E (1948) The influence of alterations in posture of the limbs on cortically induced movements. Brain 71:26–33

6 The Scapula and Pelvis

6.1 Introduction

The pelvic girdle and the shoulder girdle are not alike in their functions related to stabilization and motion of the extremities. In the shoulder girdle the scapula and clavicle work together as unit. The scapula's primary support is muscles with only one attachment to the axial skeleton, at the manubrium. The shoulder girdle is dependent on muscular function and its ability to adjust to the underlying rib cage. In its normal function it is not a weight-bearing structure. The scapula patterns are activated (whether for motion or stabilization) within the upper extremity patterns and all the upper extremity patterns and scapula motions integrate together.

The pelvic girdle, consisting of the sacrum and the innominate or coxal (hip) bone, is directly attached to the spine and is dependent mostly on vertebral support. It is a weight bearing structure. The pelvic patterns do not always function in accord with the lower extremity patterns because the pelvis is truly divided in its function. The sacrum is an extension of the lumbar spine and functions in accordance with spinal function. It is only involved in lower extremity function as an extension of the innominate. The innominate bone is clearly an extension of the lower extremity and in the efficient state moves with each lower extremity component. The Sacro-iliac (SI) articulation is the transition between the axial skeleton and the lower extremity. Therefore, the pelvic patterns are directed through the sacrum to the lumbar spine while the lower extremity patterns extend into the pelvic girdle through the innominate. The lower extremity motions are supported and complimented, whether in weight bearing or non-weight bearing, by innominate motions. The sacrum has the functional role in the pelvic patterns. The innominate has only a minor passive function unless the extremity is added. That is why, for example, it is so important to proceed to rolling as soon as the pelvic pattern is developed (G. Johnson 1999).

6.2 Applications

Exercise of the scapula and pelvis is important for treatment of the neck, the trunk, and the extremities. The scapular muscles control or influence the function of the cervical and thoracic spine. Proper function of the upper extremities requires both motion and stability of the scapula. Pelvic motion and stability are required for proper function of the trunk and the lower extremities.

Exercise of the scapula and pelvis can have various goals:

THERAPEUTIC GOALS ▬▬▬▬▬▬▬▬▬▬▬▬▬▬▬▬▬

- **Scapula**
  - ▶ Exercise the scapula independently for motion and stability.
  - ▶ Exercise trunk muscles by using timing for emphasis and resistance for facilitation.
  - ▶ Exercise functional activities such as rolling.
  - ▶ Facilitate cervical motion and stability (by resisting scapular motion and stabilization, since the scapula and neck reinforce each other).
  - ▶ Facilitate arm motion and stability (by resisting scapular motion and stabilization, since the scapula and arm muscles reinforce each other).
  - ▶ Treat the lower trunk indirectly through irradiation
- **Pelvis**
  - ▶ Exercise the pelvis for motion and stability.
  - ▶ Facilitate trunk motion and stability.
  - ▶ Exercise functional activities such as rolling.
  - ▶ Facilitate leg motion and stability.
  - ▶ Treat the upper trunk and cervical areas indirectly through irradiation.

6.3 Basic Procedures

Diagonal Motion

The scapular and pelvic patterns occur in two diagonals: anterior elevation – posterior depression and posterior elevation – anterior depression. Movement in the diagonals is an arc that follows the curve of the patient's torso. When the scapula or pelvis is moved within the diagonal, the patient will not roll forward or back or rotate around one spinal segment.

Picture a patient lying on the left side (Fig. 6.1). Now imagine a clock with the 12 o'clock position toward the patient's head, the 6 o'clock position toward the feet, the 3 o'clock position anterior and the 9 o'clock position posterior. When working with the right scapula or pelvis, anterior elevation is toward 1 o'clock and posterior depression toward 7 o'clock. Posterior elevation is toward 11 o'clock and anterior depression toward 5 o'clock (Fig. 6.1).

Now imagine that the patient is lying on the right side. The 12 o'clock position is still toward the patient's head but the 3 o'clock position is posterior and the 9 o'clock position anterior. Working with the left scapula or pelvis, anterior elevation is toward 11 o'clock and posterior depression toward 5 o'clock; posterior – elevation is toward 1 o'clock and anterior depression toward 7 o'clock. In this chapter we show all patterns being done on the patient's left scapula or pelvis. All references are to motion of the left scapula or the left side of the pelvis.

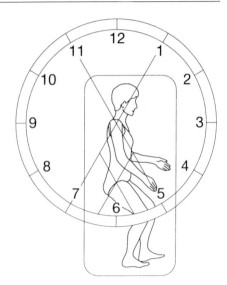

Fig. 6.1. Diagonal motion

Patient Position

We illustrate the basic scapula and pelvic patterns with the patient side lying on a treatment table. The use of these patterns in other positions is illustrated in later chapters.

The procedures start with the patient in a stable side lying position, the hips and knees flexed as much as the activity needs to get an optimal result. The patient should be positioned so that his or her back is close to the edge of the treatment table. The patient's spine is maintained in a normal alignment and the head and neck in as neutral a position as possible, neither flexed nor extended. The patient's head is supported in line with the spine, avoiding lateral bend.

Before beginning a scapula or pelvis pattern, place the scapula or pelvis in a mid-position where the line of the two diagonals cross. The scapula should not be rotated, and the glenohumeral complex should lie in the antero-posterior midline. The pelvis should be in the middle, between anterior and posterior tilt. You can use a pillow between the knees when the pelvis is rotated. From this midline position, the scapula or pelvis can then be moved into the elongated range of the pattern.

Therapist Position

The therapist stands behind the patient, facing the line of the scapular or pelvic diagonal and with arms and hand aligned with the motion. All the grips described in this chapter assume that the therapist is in this position.

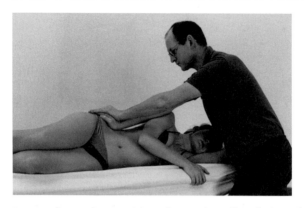

Fig. 6.2. Alternative position: the therapist is in front of the patient (anterior elevation of the pelvis)

In an alternative position the patient lies facing the edge of the treatment table. The therapist stands in front of the patient in the line of the chosen diagonal. The hand placement on the patient's body remains the same but the grips use different areas of the therapist's hands (Fig. 6.2).

The scapular and pelvic patterns can also be done with the patient lying on the mats. In this position, the therapist must kneel on the mats either in front of or behind the patient. Weight shifting is done by moving from the position of sitting on the heels (kneeling down) to partial or fully upright kneeling (kneeling up).

Grips

The grips follow the basic procedure for manual contact, that is opposite the direction of movement. This section describes the two-handed grips used when the patient is side lying and the therapist is standing behind the patient. These grips are modified when the therapist's or patient's position is changed, and some modification is also needed when the therapist can use only one hand while the other hand controls another pattern or extremity.

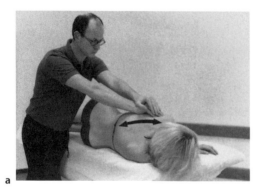

a

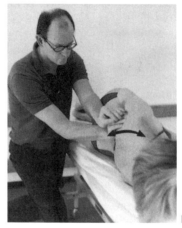

b

Fig. 6.3 a, b. The direction of the resistance is an arc (posterior depression of the scapula)

Resistance

The direction of the resistance is an arc following the contour of the patient's body. The angle of the therapist's hands and arms changes as the scapula or pelvis moves through this arc of diagonal motion (Fig. 6.3).

6.4 Scapular Diagonals

6.4.1 Specific Scapula Patterns

Scapula patterns can be done with the patient lying on the treatment table, on mats, sitting, or standing. The humerus must be free to move as the scapula moves. Side lying (illustrated) allows free motion of the scapula and easy reinforcement of trunk activities. The main muscle components are as follows (extrapolated from Kendall and McCreary 1983). We know of no confirming electromyographic studies.

Table 6.1 Movement

Movement	Muscles: principal components
Anterior elevation	Levator scapulae, rhomboids, serratus anterior
Posterior depression	Serratus anterior (lower), rhomboids, latissimus dorsi
Posterior elevation	Trapezius, levator scapulae
Anterior depression	Rhomboids, serratus anterior, pectoralis minor and major

Anterior Elevation and Posterior Depression (Fig. 6.4 a–c)

The therapist stands behind the patient, facing up toward the patient's head.

Anterior Elevation (Figs. 6.4 b, 6.5):

Grip. Place one hand on the anterior aspect of the glenohumeral joint and the acromion with your fingers cupped. The other hand covers and supports the first. Contact is with the fingers and not the palm of the hand.

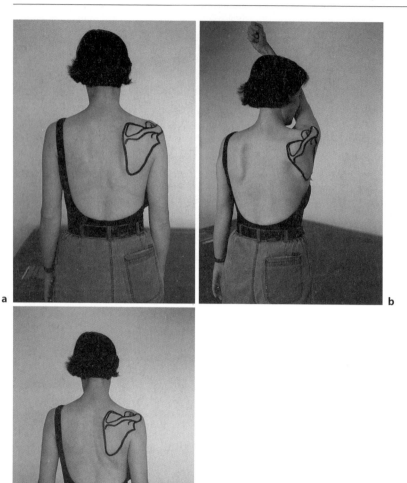

Fig. 6.4 a–c. Scapula diagonal: anterior elevation/posterior depression. **a** Neutral position; **b** anterior elevation; **c** posterior depression

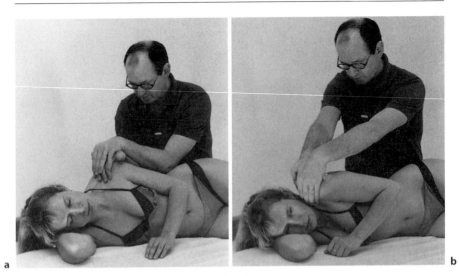

a   b

Fig. 6.5 a, b. Resistance to scapular anterior elevation

Elongated Position (Fig. 6.5 a). Pull the entire scapula down and back toward the lower thoracic spine (posterior depression). Be sure that the glenohumeral complex is positioned posterior to the central anteroposterior line of the body (mid-frontal plane). You should see and feel that the anterior muscles of the neck are taut. Do not pull so far that you lift the patient's head up. Continued pressure on the scapula should not cause the patient to roll back or rotate the spine around one segment.

Command. "Shrug your shoulder up toward your nose." "Pull".

Movement. The scapula moves up and forward in a line aimed approximately at the patient's nose.

Body Mechanics. Keep your arms relaxed and let your body give the resistance by shifting your weight from the back to the front leg.

Resistance. The line of resistance is an arc following the curve of the patient's body. Start with your elbows low and your forearms parallel to the patient's back. At the end of the pattern your elbows are extending and you are lifting upward.

End Position (Fig. 6.5 b). The scapula is up and forward with the acromion close to the patient's nose. The scapular retractor and depressor muscles are taut.

Posterior Depression (Fig. 6.4 c, 6.6)

Grip. Place the heels of your hands along the vertebral border of the scapula with one hand just above (cranial to) the other. Your fingers lie on the scapula pointing toward the acromion. Try to keep all pressure below (caudal to) the spine of the scapula.

Elongated Position (Fig. 6.6 a). Push the scapula up and forward (Anterior elevation) until you feel and see that the posterior muscles below the spine of the scapula are tight. Continued pressure should not cause the patient to roll forward or rotate the spine around one segment.

Command. "Push your shoulder blade down to me." "Push".

Movement. The scapula moves down (caudal) and back (adduction), toward the lower thoracic spine.

Body Mechanics. Flex your elbows to keep your forearms parallel to the line of resistance. Shift your weight to your back foot and allow your elbows to drop as the patient's scapula moves down and back (Fig. 6.6b).

Resistance. The line of resistance is an arc following the curve of the patient's body. Start by lifting the scapula down toward the patient's nose. As the scapula moves toward the anteroposterior midline, the resistance is forward and almost parallel to the supporting table. By the end of the motion the resistance is forward and upward toward the ceiling.

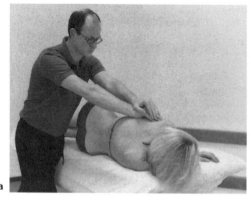
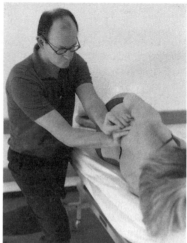

a

Fig. 6.6 a, b. Resistance to scapular posterior depression

b

End Position (Fig. 6.6b). The scapula is depressed and retracted with the glenohumeral complex posterior to the central anteroposterior line of the trunk. The vertebral border should lie flat and not wing out.

Anterior Depression and Posterior Elevation (Fig. 6.7a–c)

The therapist stands behind the patient's head facing towards the patient's bottom (right) hip.

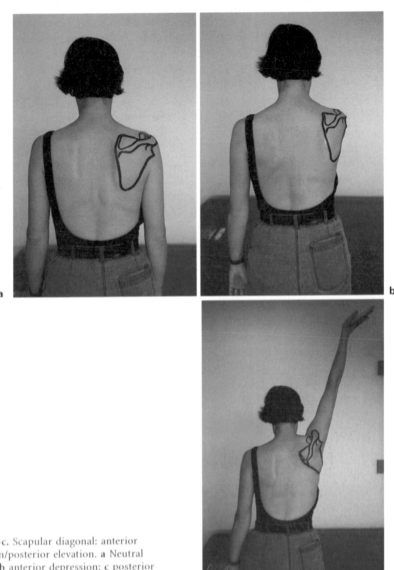

Fig. 6.7a–c. Scapular diagonal: anterior depression/posterior elevation. a Neutral position; b anterior depression; c posterior elevation

Anterior Depression (Fig. 6.7b, Fig. 6.8)

Grip. Place one hand posteriorly with the fingers holding the lateral (axillary) border of the scapula. The other hand holds anteriorly on the axillary border of the pectoralis major muscle and on the coracoid process. The fingers of both hands point toward the opposite ilium, and your arms are lined up in the same direction.

Elongated Position (Fig. 6.8a). Lift the entire scapula up and back toward the middle of the back of the head (posterior elevation). Be sure that the glenohumeral complex is positioned posterior to the central anteroposterior line of the body (mid-frontal plane). You should see and feel that the abdominal area is taut from the ipsilateral ribs to the contralateral pelvis. Continued pressure on the scapula should not cause the patient to roll back or rotate the spine around one segment.

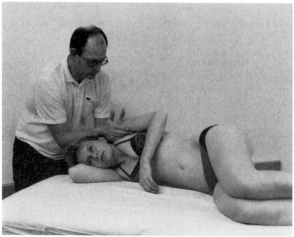

a

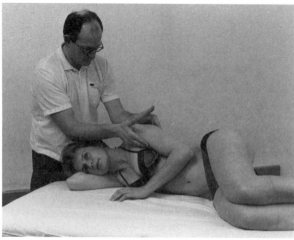

b

Fig. 6.8a, b. Resistance to scapular anterior depression

Command. "Pull your shoulder blade down toward your navel." "Pull."

Movement. The scapula moves down and forward, in a line aimed at the opposite anterior iliac crest.

Body Mechanics. Let the resistance come from your body weight as you shift from the back to the front leg.

Resistance. The resistance follows the curve of the patient's body. At the end of the pattern you are lifting in a line parallel to the front of the patient's thorax.

End Position (Fig. 6.8 b). The scapula is rotated forward, depressed, and abducted. The glenohumeral complex is anterior to the central antero-posterior line of the body.

Posterior Elevation (Fig. 6.7 c, Fig. 6.9)

Grip. Place your hands posterior on the upper trapezius muscle, staying above (superior to) the spine of the scapula. Overlap your hands as necessary to stay distal to the junction of the spine and first rib.

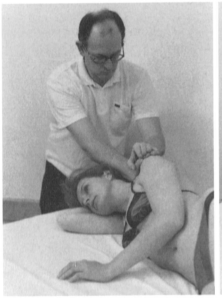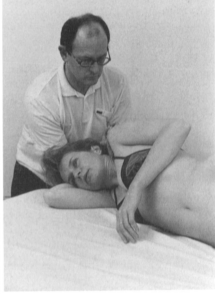

a   b

Fig. 6.9 a, b. Resistance to scapular posterior elevation

Elongated Position (Fig. 6.9 a). Round the scapula down and forward toward the opposite ilium (anterior depression) until you feel that the upper trapezius muscle is taut. Do not push so far that you lift the patient's head up. Continued pressure should not cause the patient to roll forward or rotate the spine around one segment.

Command. "Shrug your shoulder up." "Push".

Movement. The scapula shrugs up (cranially) and back (adduction) in a line aimed at the middle of the top of the patient's head. The glenohumeral complex moves posteriorly and rotates upward.

Body Mechanics. Shift your weight from the front to the back foot as the scapula moves. Your forearms stay parallel to the line of resistance.

Resistance. The resistance follows the curve of the patient's body. At the end of the pattern you are lifting around the thorax and away from top of the patient's head.

End Position (Fig. 6.9 b). The scapula is elevated and adducted, the gleno-humeral complex is posterior to the central anteroposterior line of the body.

→ **Points to remember**
- When doing pure scapular patterns the trunk does not roll or rotate.
- The glenohumeral complex is part of the scapular pattern. The humerus must be free to move along.

6.4.2 Specific Uses for Scapular Patterns

- Exercise the scapula for motion and stability (Fig. 6.10)
- Exercise trunk muscles
  - ▶ Using timing for emphasis, prevent scapular motion at the beginning of the range until you feel and see the trunk muscles contract. When this occurs, change the resistance at the scapula so that both the scapula and the trunk motion are resisted.
  - ▶ At the end of the scapular range of motion, "lock in" the scapula with a stabilizing contraction and exercise the trunk with repeated contractions.
  - ▶ Use Reversal of Antagonist techniques to train coordination and prevent or reduce fatigue of the scapular and trunk muscles.
- Exercise functional activities such as rolling.
  - ▶ When the trunk muscles are contracting you can extend their action into such functional activities as rolling forward or backward (see Sect.

11.5.1). Give a movement command such as "roll forward" and resist the functional activity using the stabilized scapula as the handle.

▶ Repeated Contractions of the functional activity will reinforce both learning the activity and the physical ability to do it.

- Facilitate cervical motion and stability (by resisting scapular motion and stabilization, since the scapula and neck reinforce each other)

  ▶ Resist the moving or stabilizing contraction at the scapula and head simultaneously to exercise the muscles that go from the cervical spine to the scapula.

  ▶ To stretch these muscles for increased range of motion, stabilize the cervical spine and resist the appropriate scapular motion.

- Facilitate arm motion and stability (by resisting scapular motion and stabilization, since the scapula and arm muscles reinforce each other). (Fig. 6.10)

  ▶ Scapular elevation patterns work with arm flexion patterns.

  ▶ Scapular depression patterns work with arm extension patterns.

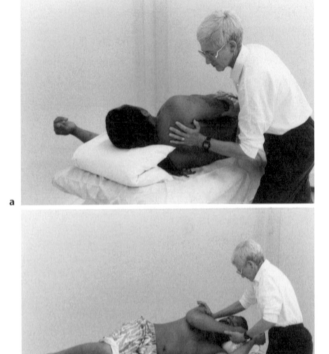

Fig. 6.10a,b. Patient with right hemiplegia. a Combination of scapula (posterior depression) with arm motion. b Combination of scapula (anterior elevation) with arm motion

- Treat the lower trunk indirectly through irradiation. Give sustained maximal resistance to stabilizing or isometric scapula patterns until you see and feel contraction of the desired lower trunk muscles.

→ **Points to remember**
- **The scapular patterns work directly on the spine as well.**
- **When using scapular patterns for rolling, the scapula is the handle and the rolling is exercised.**

6.5 Pelvic Diagonals

6.5.1 Specific Pelvic Patterns

The pelvis is part of the trunk, so the range of motion in the pelvic patterns depends on the amount of motion in the lower spine. We treat pelvic patterns as isolated from the trunk if no increased lumbar flexion or extension occurs. Pelvic patterns can be done with the patient lying, sitting, quadruped, or standing. The side that is moving must not be weight-bearing. Side lying (illustrated) allows free motion of the pelvis and easy reinforcement of trunk and lower extremity activities.

The movements and muscle components mainly involved are as follows (Kendall and McCready 1983):

Table 6.2

Movement	Muscles: principal components
Anterior elevation	Internal and external oblique abdominal muscles
Posterior depression	Contralateral Internal and external oblique abdominal muscles
Posterior elevation	Ipsilateral quadratus lumborum, ipsilateral latissimus dorsi, iliocostalis lumborum, and longissimus thoracis
Anterior depression	Contralateral quadratus lumborum, iliocostalis lumborum, and longissimus thoracis

Anterior Elevation and Posterior Depression (Fig. 6.11 a–e)

The therapist stands behind the patient facing up toward the patient's lower (right) shoulder.

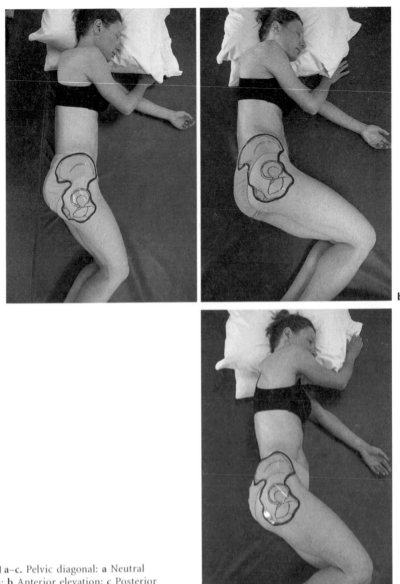

Fig. 6.11 a–c. Pelvic diagonal: **a** Neutral position; **b** Anterior elevation; **c** Posterior depression

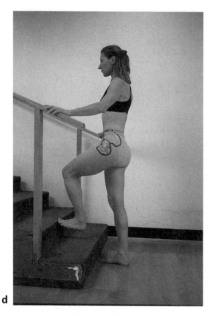
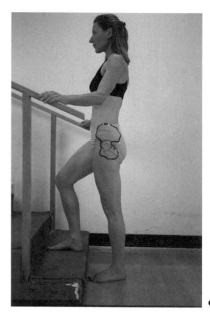

d   e

Fig. 6.11 d, e. Pelvic patterns in function: **d** pelvic pattern in anterior elevation, **e** pelvic pattern in posterior depression

Anterior Elevation (Fig. 6.11 b, d; Fig. 6.12)

Grip. The fingers of one hand grip around the crest of the ilium, on and just anterior to the midline. Your other hand overlaps the first.

Elongated Position (Fig. 6.12 a). Pull the crest of the pelvis back and down in the direction of posterior depression. See and feel that the tissues stretching from the crest of the ilium to the opposite rib cage are taut. Continued pressure should not cause the patient to roll backward or rotate the spine around one segment.

Command. "Shrug your pelvis up." "Pull."

Movement. The pelvis moves up and forward without posterior or anterior tilt. There is an anterior shortening of the trunk on that side (lateral flexion).

Body Mechanics. Start with your elbows flexed to pull the iliac crest down as well as back. As the movement progresses your elbows extend and your weight shifts from your back to your front foot.

Resistance. The line of resistance curves following the patient's body. Start by pulling the pelvis back toward you and down toward the table. As the

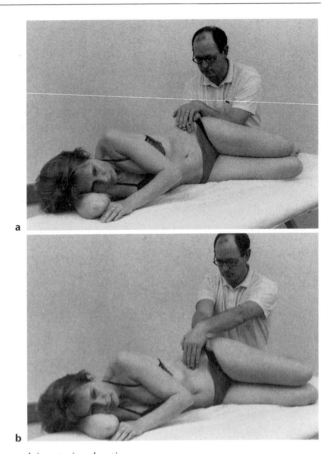

Fig. 6.12 a, b. Resistance to pelvic anterior elevation

pelvis moves to the mid-position the line of the resistance is almost straight back. At the end of the motion the resistance is up toward the ceiling.

End Position (Fig. 6.12 b). The pelvis is up (elevated) and forward (anterior) toward the lower shoulder with no increase in the anterior or posterior tilt. The upper side (left) of the trunk is shortened and laterally flexed with no change in lumbar lordosis.

Posterior Depression (Fig. 6.11 c,e; Fig. 6.13)

Grip. Place the heel of one hand on the ischial tuberosity. Overlap and reinforce the hold with your other hand. The fingers of both hands point diagonally forward.

Elongated Position (Fig. 6.13 a). Push the ischial tuberosity up and forward to bring the iliac crest down closer to the opposite rib cage (anterior elevation). Continued pressure should not cause the patient to roll forward or rotate the spine around one segment.

Command. "Sit into my hand." "Push."

Movement. The pelvis moves down and posteriorly without tilt. There is an elongation of the trunk on that side without a change in the lumbar lordosis.

Body Mechanics. Your elbows flex as the patient's pelvis moves downward and you shift your weight from your front to your back foot.

Resistance. The resistance is always upward on the ischial tuberosity while pushing diagonally forward (anterior and cranial).

End Position (Fig. 6.13 b). The pelvis is down and back (posterior) with no increase in the anterior or posterior tilt. The upper side (left) of the trunk is elongated with no change in the lumbar lordosis.

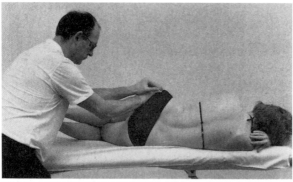

a

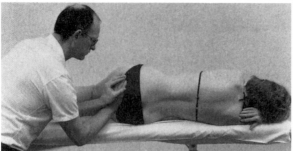

b

Fig. 6.13 a, b. Resistance to pelvic posterior depression

Anterior Depression and Posterior Elevation (Fig. 6.15 a–c)

The therapist stands behind the patient, facing toward a line representing about 25° of flexion of the patient's bottom (right) leg.

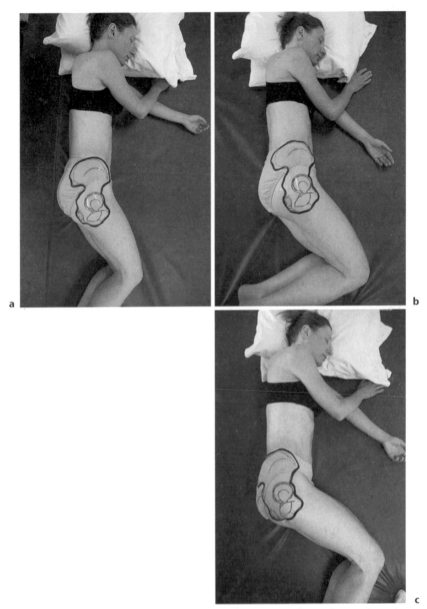

Fig. 6.14a–e. Pelvic diagonal. a Neutral position; b Anterior depression; c Posterior elevation

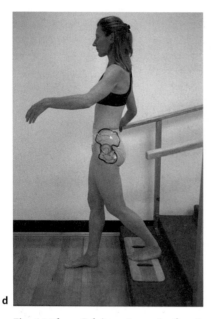
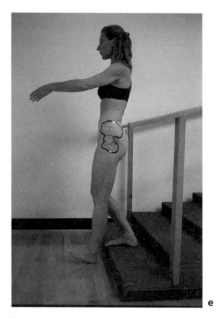

d   e

Fig. 6.14d, e. Pelvic patterns in function: **d** pelvic pattern posterior elevation, **e** pelvic pattern anterior depression

Anterior Depression (Fig. 6.14b, e; Fig. 6.15a–c)

Grip. Place the fingers of one hand on the greater trochanter of the femur. The other hand may reinforce the first hand (Fig. 6.15a) or you may grip below the anterior inferior iliac spine.

Alternate Grip. The fingers of the posterior hand grip the ischial tuberosity. The anterior hand grips below the anterior inferior iliac spine.

For a grip using the leg, place your right hand on the patient's anterior-inferior iliac spine and your left hand on the patient's left knee (Fig. 6.15b, c) You must move the patient's leg until the femur is in the line of the pattern (about 20° of hip flexion) (Fig. 6.15b).

Elongated Position (Fig. 6.15a, b). Gently move the pelvis up (cranial) and back (dorsal) toward the lower thoracic spine (posterior elevation). Be careful not to rotate or compress spinal joints.

Command. "Pull down and forward." ("Push your knee into my hand.")

Movement. The pelvis moves down and anteriorly without tilt. There is an elongation of the trunk on that side without a change in the lumbar lordosis.

Body Mechanics. Start with your elbows flexed to keep your forearms parallel to the patients back. Shift your weight to your front foot during the motion and allow your elbows to extend.

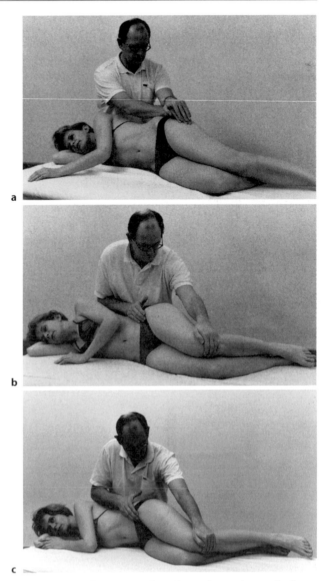

Fig. 6.15 a–c. Resistance to pelvic anterior depression. The grip on the trochanter is shown in a

Resistance. At the beginning of the movement the resistance is toward the patient's lower thoracic spine. As the motion continues, the line of the resistance follows the curve of the body. At the end of the pattern the resistance is diagonally back toward you and up toward the ceiling.

End Position (Fig. 6.15 c). The pelvis is down and forward with no increase in the anterior or posterior tilt. The trunk is elongated with no change in the lumbar lordosis.

Posterior Elevation (Fig. 6.14 c, d; Fig. 6.16)

Grip. Put the heel of one hand on the crest of the ilium, on and just posterior to the midline. Your other hand overlaps the first. There is no finger contact.

Elongated Position (Fig. 6.16 a). Gently push the pelvis down and forward until you feel and see that the posterior lateral tissues on that side are taut (anterior depression). Continued pressure should not cause the patient to roll forward or rotate the spine around one segment.

Command. "Push your pelvis up and back – gently."

Movement. The pelvis moves up and back without tilt. There is a posterior shortening of the trunk on that side (lateral flexion).

Body Mechanics. As the pelvis moves up and back shift your weight to your back foot. At the same time flex and drop your elbows so that they point down toward the table.

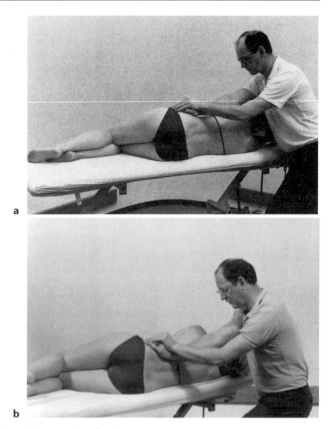

Fig. 6.16 a, b. Resistance to pelvic posterior elevation

Resistance. The resistance begins by lifting the posterior iliac crest around toward the front of the table. At the end of the motion the resistance has made an arc around the body and is now lifting the ilia crest up toward the ceiling.

End Position (Fig. 6.16b). The pelvis is up and back with no increase in the anterior or posterior tilt. The upper side (left) of the trunk is shortened and laterally flexed with no increase in lumbar lordosis.

Figure 6.17a,b shows a pelvic diagonal used when treating a patient with hemiplegia.

→ **Points to remember**
- Pure pelvic patterns do not change the amount of pelvic tilt.
- The pelvic motion comes from activity of the trunk muscles. Do not allow the leg to push the pelvis up.
- The muscles involved in pelvic depression are the contralateral pelvic elevating muscles.

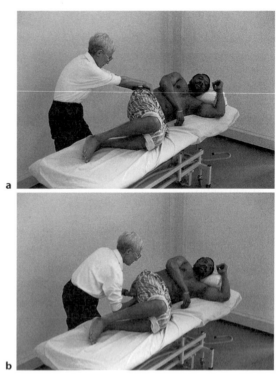

Fig. 6.17 a, b. Patient with right hemiplegia. a Resistance to pelvic anterior elevation. b Resistance to pelvic posterior depression

6.5.2 Specific Uses for Pelvic Patterns

The pelvis and lower extremities facilitate and reinforce each other. Pelvic depression patterns work with and facilitate weight-bearing motions of the legs. Pelvic elevation patterns work with and facilitate stepping or leg lifting motions.

- Exercise the pelvis for motion and stability. (Fig. 6.17 a,b)
- Facilitate trunk motion and stability by using timing for emphasis and resistance for facilitation.
  - ▶ Resist the pelvic patterns to exercise lower trunk flexor, extensor, and lateral flexor muscles The pelvis should not move further into an anterior or posterior tilt during these exercise.
    1) Use Repeated Stretch from beginning of range or through range to strengthen these trunk muscles.
    2) Use Reversal of Antagonist techniques to train coordination and prevent or reduce fatigue of the working muscles.
  - ▶ Use Stabilizing Reversals or Rhythmic Stabilization to facilitate lower trunk and pelvic stability.
- Exercise functional trunk activities.
  - ▶ Use a stabilizing contraction to lock in the pelvis, then give a functional command such as "roll" and resist the activity using the stabilized pelvis as the handle (see Sect. 11.3.1).
  - ▶ Use Repeated Contractions to strengthen and reinforce learning of the functional activity.
  - ▶ Use the technique Combination of Isotonics to teach control of the trunk motions. Have the patient control trunk motion with concentric and eccentric contractions while maintaining the pelvic stabilization.
  - ▶ Use reversal techniques to prevent or relieve muscular fatigue.
- The pelvis and lower extremities facilitate and reinforce each other.
  - ▶ Pelvic depression patterns work with and facilitate weight-bearing motions of the legs. Lock in pelvic posterior depression then exercise extension motions of the ipsilateral lower extremity.
  - ▶ Pelvic elevation patterns work with and facilitate stepping or leg lifting motions. Lock in pelvic anterior elevation then exercise flexion motions of the ipsilateral lower extremity.
- Treat the upper trunk and cervical areas indirectly through irradiation. Give sustained maximal resistance to stabilizing or isometric pelvic patterns until you see and feel contraction of the desired upper trunk and cervical muscles.

→ **Points to remember**
- **Pelvic motions work with and facilitate the leg motions, pelvic patterns do not correspond exactly with lower extremity patterns.**
- **When using pelvic patterns for rolling, the pelvis is the handle and the rolling is exercised.**

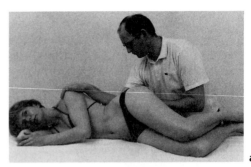

a

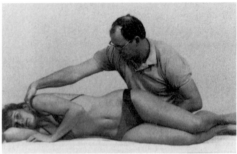

Fig. 6.18 a, b. Symmetrical-reciprocal exercise: the scapula moves in anterior elevation, the pelvis in posterior depression

b

6.6 Symmetrical, Reciprocal and Asymmetrical Exercises

In addition to the exercises carried out with one body part in one direction (the scapula moving into anterior elevation) and in both directions (the scapula moving back and forth between anterior elevation and posterior depression), both scapulae or the scapula and pelvis can be exercised simultaneously. Any combination of scapular and pelvic patterns may be used, limited only by the patient's abilities and the therapist's imagination. Here we describe and illustrate two combinations. Use the basic procedures (grip, command, resistance, timing, etc.) and techniques when you use the symmetrical and asymmetrical pattern combinations just as when you work with single patterns in one direction.

6.6.1 Symmetrical-Reciprocal Exercise

Here the scapula and pelvis move in the same diagonal but in opposite patterns (Figs. 6.18, 6.19, 6.20). You position your body parallel to the lines of the diagonals.

This combination of scapular and pelvic motions results in full trunk elongation and shortening with counter rotation. The motion is an enlarged version of the normal motion of scapula, pelvis and trunk during walking.

Scapular anterior elevation-pelvic posterior depression (Fig. 6.18.) Scapular posterior depression-Pelvic anterior elevation (Fig. 6.20). Trunk extension with rotation using a symmetrical combination of scapula anterior elevation with pelvic posterior depression with extremity motion (Fig. 6.19).

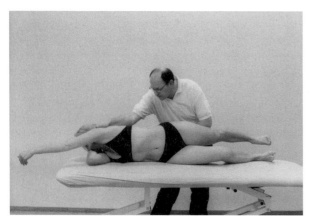

Fig. 6.19. Trunk extension with rotation: symmetrical reciprocal combination of scapula and pelvis with extremity motion

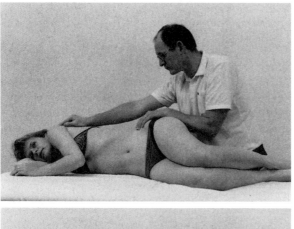

a

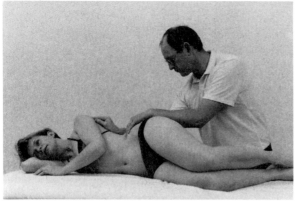

b

Fig. 6.20 a, b. Symmetrical-reciprocal exercise: the scapula moves in posterior depression, the pelvis in anterior elevation

6.6.2 Asymmetrical Exercise

In this combination the scapula and pelvis move in opposite diagonals and the diagonals are not parallel. (Figs. 6.21, 6.22) Position your body in the middle and align your forearms so that one is in the line of each diagonal. You cannot use your body weight for resistance with this combination.

When both the scapula and pelvis move in the anterior patterns (forward toward each other) the result is mass trunk flexion. (Fig. 6.21, Fig. 6.23) When both move in the posterior patterns (backward away from each) other) the result is mass trunk extension with elongation (Fig. 6.22).

Fig. 6.24 shows asymmetrical and symmetrical combinations used with a patient with hemiplegia.

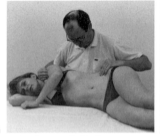 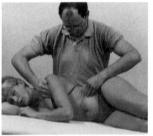

Fig. 6.21. Asymmetrical exercise for trunk flexion: the scapula moves in anterior depression, the pelvis in anterior elevation

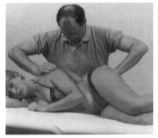 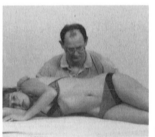

Fig. 6.22. Asymmetrical exercise for trunk extension: the scapula moves in posterior elevation, the pelvis in posterior depression

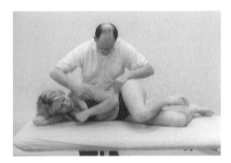

Fig. 6.23. Trunk flexion: Asymmetrical combination of scapula and pelvis with extremity motion

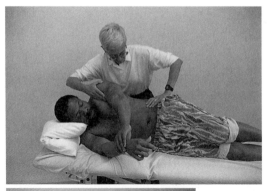

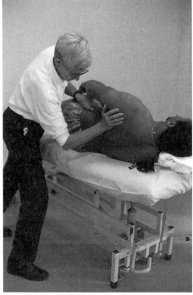

Fig. 6.24a,b. Patient with right hemiplegia. **a** Mass trunk flexion: combination of scapular anterior depression and pelvic anterior elevation. **b** Trunk rotation: combination of scapular posterior depression and pelvic anterior elevation

Reference

Johnson, G (1999) personal communication
Kendall FP, McCreary EK (1983) Muscles, testing and function. Williams and Wilkins, Baltimore

7 The Upper Extremity

7.1 Introduction and Basic Procedures

Upper extremity patterns are used to treat dysfunction caused by neurologic problems, muscular disorders or joint restrictions. These patterns are also used to exercise the trunk. Resistance to strong arm muscles produces irradiation to weaker muscles elsewhere in the body.

We can use all the techniques with the arm patterns. The choice of individual techniques or combinations of techniques will depend on the patient's condition and the treatment goals. You can, for instance, combine Dynamic Reversals with Combination of Isotonics, Repeated Contractions with Dynamic Reversals, or, Contract-Relax or Hold-Relax with Combination of Isotonics and Dynamic Reversals.

Diagonal Motion

The upper extremity has two diagonals:
1. Flexion–abduction–external rotation and extension–adduction–internal rotation
2. Flexion–adduction–external rotation and extension–abduction–internal rotation

The shoulder and the wrist-hand complex are tied together in the pattern synergy. The elbow is free to move into flexion, move into extension, or remain motionless. Do not allow the arm to move laterally out of the groove to compensate for any limitation of shoulder motion.

Scapular motion is an integral part of each pattern. For a description of the motions making up the scapular patterns see Chapter 6.

The basic patterns of the left arm with the subject supine are shown in Fig. 7.1. All descriptions refer to this arrangement. To work with the right arm just change the word "left" to "right" in the instructions. Variations of position are shown later in the chapter.

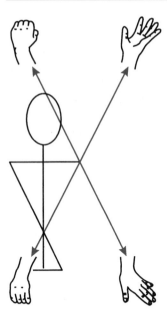

Fig. 7.1. Upper extremity diagonals
(Courtesy of V. Jung)

Patient Position

! Note: Position the patient close to the left edge of the table.

Support the patient's head and neck in a comfortable position, as close to
neutral as possible. Before beginning an upper extremity pattern, visualize
the patient's arm in a middle position where the lines of the two diagonals
cross. Starting with the shoulder and forearm in neutral rotation, move the
extremity into the elongated range of the pattern with the proper rotation,
beginning with the wrist and fingers.

Therapist Position

! Note: The therapist stands on the left side of the table facing the line of the
diagonal, arms and hands aligned with the motion.

All grips described in the first part of each section assume that the therapist
is in this position.

We give the basic position and body mechanics for exercising the straight
arm pattern. When we describe variations in the patterns we identify any
changes in position or body mechanics. The therapist's position can vary
within the guidelines for the basic procedures. Some of these variations are
illustrated at the end of the chapter.

Grips

The grips follow the basic procedures for manual contact, opposite the direction of movement. The first part of this chapter (Section 7.2) describes the two-handed grip used when the therapist stands next to the moving upper extremity. The basic grip is described for each straight arm pattern. The grips are modified when the therapist's or patient's position is changed. The grips also change when the therapist can use only one hand while the other hand controls another extremity. The grip on the hand contacts the active surface, dorsal or palmar, and holds the sides of the hand to resist the rotary components. Using the lumbrical grip will prevent squeezing or pinching the patient's hand. Remember, pain inhibits effective motion.

We recommend distal grips when the arm patterns start straight and optimal elongation or stretch is important. If the arm and elbow go from extension to flexion, change the proximal grip from the forearm to the upper arm for better shoulder control. If the arm moves from flexion to extension, we recommend starting with the proximal grip on the humerus for better elongation of all scapula and shoulder muscles.

Resistance

The direction of the resistance is an arc back toward the starting position. The angle of the therapist's hands and arms changes as the limb moves through the pattern.

Traction and Approximation

Traction and approximation are an important part of the resistance. Use traction at the beginning of the motion in both flexion and extension. Use approximation at the end of the range to stabilize the arm and scapula.

Normal Timing and Timing for Emphasis

Normal Timing

The hand and wrist (distal component) begin the pattern, moving through their full range. Rotation at the shoulder and forearm accompanies the rotation (radial or ulnar deviation) of the wrist. After the distal movement is completed, the scapula moves together with the shoulder or shoulder and elbow through their range. The arm moves through the diagonals in a straight line with rotation occurring smoothly throughout the motion.

Timing for Emphasis

In the sections on timing for emphasis we offer some suggestions for exercising components of the patterns. Any of the techniques may be used. We have found that Repeated Stretch (Repeated Contractions) and Combination of Isotonics work well. Do not limit yourself to the exercises we suggest in this section, use your imagination.

Stretch

In the arm patterns we use stretch-stimulus with or without the stretch-reflex to facilitate an easier or stronger movement, or to start the motion.

Repeated Stretch (Repeated Contractions) during the motion facilitates a stronger motion or guides the motion into the desired direction. Repeated Stretch at the beginning of the pattern is used when the patient has difficulty initiating the motion and to guide the direction of the motion. To get the stretch reflex the therapist must elongate both the distal and proximal components. Be sure you do not overstretch a muscle or put too much tension on joint structure. This is particularly important with the wrist joint

Irradiation and Reinforcement

We can use strong arm patterns (single or bilateral) to get irradiation into all other parts of our body. The patient's position in combination with the amount of resistance controls the amount of irradiation. We use this irradiation to strengthen muscles or mobilize joints in other parts of the body, to relax muscle chains, and to facilitate a functional activity such as rolling.

7.2 **Flexion–Abduction–External Rotation** (Fig. 7.2)

Joint	Movement	Muscles: principal components (Kendall and McCreary 1983)
Scapula	Posterior elevation	Trapezius, levator scapulae, serratus anterior
Shoulder	Flexion, abduction, external rotation	Deltoid (anterior), biceps (long head), coracobrachialis, supraspinatus, infraspinatus, teres minor
Elbow	Extended (position unchanged)	Triceps, anconeus
Forearm	Supination	Biceps, brachioradialis, supinator
Wrist	Radial extension	Extensor carpi radialis (longus and brevis)
Fingers	Extension, radial deviation	Extensor digitorum longus, interossei
Thumb	Extension, abduction	Extensor pollicis (longus and brevis), abductor pollicis longus

Grip

Distal Hand

Your right hand grips the dorsal surface of the patient's hand. Your fingers are on the radial side (1st and 2nd metacarpal), your thumb gives counter-pressure on the ulnar border (5th metacarpal). There is no contact on the palm.

 Caution: Do not squeeze the hand.

Proximal Hand

From underneath the arm, hold the radial and ulnar sides of the patient's forearm proximal to the wrist. The lumbrical grip allows you to avoid placing any pressure on the anterior (palmar) surface of the forearm.

Alternative Grip

To emphasize shoulder or scapula motions, move the proximal hand to grip the upper arm or the scapula after the wrist completes its motion (Fig. 7.2 d, e).

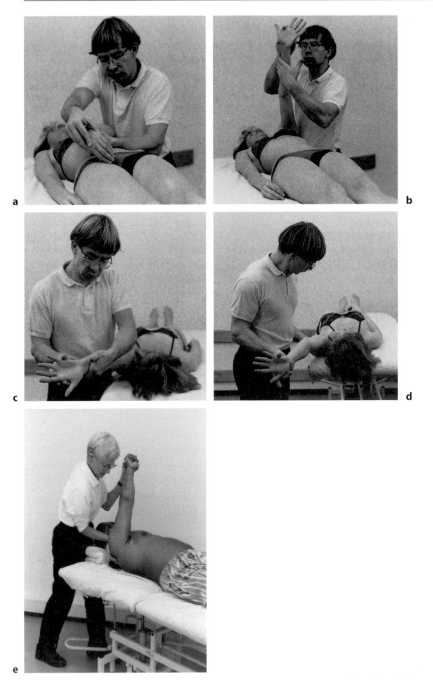

Fig. 7.2 a-e. Flexion–abduction–external rotation. **a** Starting position; **b** mid-position; **c** end position; **d** emphasizing the motion of the shoulder. **e** Patient with right hemiplegia. Flexion–abduction–external rotation: proximal hand for scapula posterior elevation and trunk elongation

Elongated Position

Place the wrist in ulnar flexion and the forearm into pronation. Maintain the wrist and hand in position while you move the shoulder into extension and adduction. You may use gentle traction to help elongate the shoulder and scapula muscles. The humerus crosses over the midline to the right and the palm faces toward the right ilium. The traction brings the scapula into anterior depression A continuation of this motion would bring the patient into trunk flexion to the right.

Body Mechanics

Stand in a stride position by or above the patient's shoulder with your left foot forward. Face the line of motion. Start with the weight on your front foot and let the patient's motion push your weight to your back foot. Continue facing the line of motion.

Stretch

Apply the stretch to the shoulder and hand simultaneously. Your proximal hand does a rapid traction with rotation of the shoulder and scapula. Your distal hand gives traction to the wrist.

 Caution: Traction the wrist in line with the metacarpal bones. Do not force the wrist into more flexion.

Command

"Hand up, lift your arm." "Lift!"

Movement

The fingers and thumb extend as the wrist moves into radial extension. The radial side of the hand leads as the shoulder moves into flexion with abduction and external rotation. The scapula moves into posterior elevation. Continuation of this motion is an upward reach with elongation of the left side of the trunk.

Resistance

Your distal hand combines traction through the extended wrist with a rotary resistance for the radial deviation. Resistance to the forearm supination and shoulder external rotation and abduction comes from the rotary resistance at the wrist. The traction force resists the motions of wrist extension and shoulder flexion.

Your proximal hand combines a traction force with rotary resistance. The line of resistance is back toward the starting position. Maintaining the traction force will guide your resistance in the proper arc.

Use approximation through the humerus at the end of the shoulder range to resist the scapula elevation and stabilize the shoulder.

End Position

The humerus is in full flexion (about three fingers from the left ear), the palm facing about 45° to the coronal (lateral) plane. The scapula is in posterior elevation. The elbow remains extended. The wrist is in full radial extension, fingers and thumb extended toward the radial side.

Timing for Emphasis

You may prevent motion in the beginning of the shoulder flexion or in the mid-range and exercise the wrist, hand, or fingers.

→ **Points to remember**
- **The stretch at the wrist is done with traction, not more flexion**
- **Too much shoulder rotation limits the scapular movement**
- **At the end of the pattern the trunk is in elongation**

7.2.1 Flexion–Abduction–External Rotation with Elbow Flexion (Fig. 7.3)

Joint	Movement	Muscles: principal components (Kendall and McCreary 1983)
Scapula	Posterior elevation	Trapezius, levator scapulae, serratus anterior
Shoulder	Flexion, abduction, external rotation	Deltoid (anterior), biceps (long head), coracobrachialis, supraspinatus, infraspinatus, teres minor
Elbow	Flexion	Biceps, brachialis
Forearm	Supination	Biceps, brachioradialis, supinator
Wrist	Radial extension	Extensor carpi radialis (longus and brevis)
Fingers	Extension, radial deviation	Extensor digitorum longus, interossei
Thumb	Extension, abduction	Extensor pollicis (longus and brevis), abductor pollicis longus

Grip

Distal Hand

Your distal grip is the same as described in Sect. 7.2 for the straight arm pattern.

Proximal Hand

Your proximal hand may start with the grip used for the straight arm pattern. As the shoulder and elbow begin to flex, move this hand up to grip the humerus. You wrap your hand around the humerus from the medial side and use your fingers to give pressure opposite the direction of motion. The resistance to rotation comes from the line of your fingers and forearm.

Alternative Grip

The proximal hand may move to the scapula to emphasize that motion.

Elongated Position

Position the limb as for the straight arm pattern.

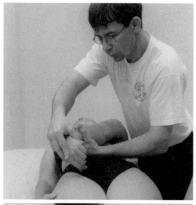

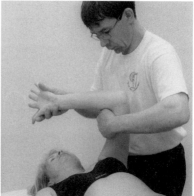

a

b

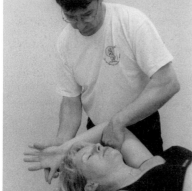

Fig. 7.3 a–f. Flexion–abduction–external rotation with elbow flexion. **a–c** Usual position of the therapist; **d, e** alternative position with therapist on the other side of the table

c

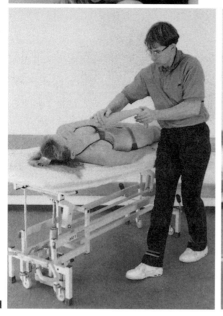

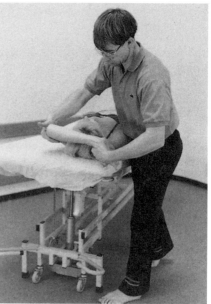

d

e

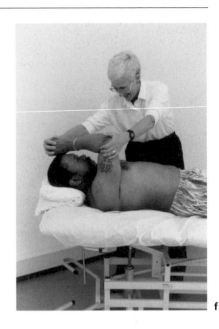

Fig. 7.3 f. Flexion–abduction–external rotation with elbow flexion. Patient with hemiplegia, the patient is asked to touch his head

f

Body Mechanics

Stand in the same stride position as for the straight arm pattern. Allow the patient to push your weight from your front to your back foot. Face the line of motion.

Alternative Position

You may stand on the right side of the table facing up toward the patient's left shoulder. Put your left hand on the patient's hand, your right hand on the humerus. Stand in a stride with your right leg forward. As the patient's arm moves up into flexion, step forward with your left leg. If you choose this position, move the patient to the right side of the table (Fig. 7.3 d, e).

Stretch

Use the same motions for the stretch reflex that you used with the straight arm pattern.

> **❗ Caution:** Traction the wrist in line with the metacarpal bones. Do not force the wrist into more flexion.

Command

"Hand up, lift your arm and bend your elbow." "Lift!"

Movement

The fingers and thumb extend and the wrist moves into radial extension as in the straight arm pattern. The elbow and shoulder motions begin next. The elbow flexion causes the hand and forearm to move across the face as the shoulder completes its flexion.

Resistance

Your distal hand resists the wrist and forearm as it did in the straight arm pattern. Add resistance to the elbow flexion by giving traction in and arc back toward the starting position.

Your proximal hand combines rotary resistance with traction through the humerus toward the starting position. Give a separate force with each hand so that the resistance is appropriate for the strength of the shoulder and elbow.

End Position

The humerus is in full flexion with the scapula in posterior elevation. The elbow is flexed, and the patient's forearm is touching the head. The wrist is again in full radial extension, fingers and thumb extended toward the radial side. The rotation in the shoulder and forearm are the same as in the straight arm pattern. If you extend the patient's elbow, the position is the same as in the straight arm pattern.

Timing for Emphasis

With three moving segments, shoulder, elbow and wrist, you may lock in any two and exercise the third.

With the elbow bent it is easy to exercise the external rotation separately from the forearm rotation, and the supination separately from the shoulder rotation. Do this exercise where the strength of the shoulder and elbow is greatest. You may work through the full range of shoulder external rotation during these exercises but return to the groove before finishing the pattern.

When exercising the patient's wrist or hand, move your proximal hand to the forearm and give resistance to the shoulder and elbow with that hand. Your distal hand is now free to give appropriate resistance to the wrist and hand motions. To exercise the fingers and thumb, move your proximal hand to give resistance just distal to the wrist. Your distal hand can now exercise the fingers, jointly or individually.

Prevent motion in the beginning or middle range of shoulder flexion and exercise the elbow, wrist, hand, or fingers.

→ **Points to remember**
- **The stretch at the wrist is done with traction, not more flexion**
- **Resist the elbow flexion with traction back to the starting position**
- **Extend the patient's elbow, the position is the same as the straight arm pattern**
- **Give a functional command such as "touch the top of your head"**

7.2.2 Flexion–Abduction–External Rotation with Elbow Extension (Fig. 7.4)

Joint	Movement	Muscles: principal components (Kendall and McCreary 1983)
Scapula	Posterior elevation	Trapezius, levator scapulae, serratus anterior
Shoulder	Flexion, abduction, external rotation	Deltoid (anterior), biceps (long head), coracobrachialis, supraspinatus, infraspinatus, teres minor
Elbow	Extension	Triceps, anconeus
Forearm	Supination	Biceps, brachioradialis, supinator
Wrist	Radial extension	Extensor carpi radialis (longus and brevis)
Fingers	Extension, radial deviation	Extensor digitorum longus, interossei
Thumb	Extension, abduction	Extensor pollicis (longus and brevis), abductor pollicis longus

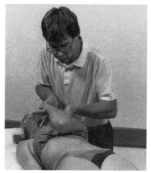 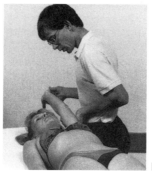

a

b

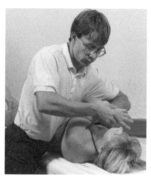

c

Fig. 7.4a–c. Flexion–abduction–external rotation with elbow extension. a, b Standard grips; c Grip variation

Grip

Your distal grip is the same as for the straight arm pattern. Wrap your proximal hand around the humerus from the medial side so that your fingers give pressure opposing the direction of motion.

Elongated Position

The position of the patient's scapula, shoulder, forearm, and wrist are the same as for the straight arm pattern. The elbow is fully flexed.

Alternative starting position (Fig. 7.4 c)

The therapist can also stand close to the pelvis, facing the patient. The left hand grips the humerus and triceps under the forearm and tractions the upper arm into extension, adduction and internal rotation and the scapula into anterior depression.

Body Mechanics

Stand in the same stride position used for the straight arm pattern. Shift your weight as you did for the straight arm pattern.

Stretch

Apply the stretch to the shoulder, elbow, and hand simultaneously. Your proximal hand stretches the shoulder and scapula with a rapid traction and rotation motion. Your distal hand continues giving traction to the hand and wrist while stretching the elbow extension.

> **!** Caution: Traction the wrist, do not force it into more flexion.

Command

"Hand up, push your arm up and straighten your elbow as you go." "Push!" "Reach up."

Movement

The fingers and thumb extend and the wrist moves into radial extension as before. The elbow and shoulder motions begin next. The elbow extension moves the hand and forearm in front of the face as the shoulder flexes. The elbow reaches full extension as the shoulder and scapula complete their motion.

Resistance

Your distal hand resists the wrist and forearm as in the straight arm pattern. Give resistance to the elbow extension by rotating the forearm and hand back toward the starting position of elbow flexion. Your proximal hand gives traction through the humerus combined with rotary resistance back toward the starting position.

Each of your hands uses the proper force to make the resistance appropriate for the strength of the elbow and the strength of the shoulder. Use approximation through the humerus at the end of the shoulder range to resist the scapula elevation and stabilize the shoulder and elbow.

End Position

The end position is the same as the straight arm pattern.

Timing for Emphasis

Prevent elbow extension at the beginning of the range and exercise the shoulder. Lock in shoulder flexion in mid-range and exercise the elbow extension with supination.

→ Points to remember
   ● The stretch at the wrist is done with traction, not more flexion
   ● Use a rotary force back into pronation to resist the elbow extension

---

7.3 **Extension–Adduction–Internal Rotation** (Fig. 7.5)

Joint	Movement	Muscles: principal components (Kendall and McCreary 1983)
Scapula	Anterior depression	Serratus anterior (lower), pectoralis minor, rhomboids
Shoulder	Extension, adduction, internal rotation	Pectoralis major, teres major, subscapularis
Elbow	Extended (position unchanged)	Triceps, anconeus
Forearm	Pronation	Brachioradialis, pronator (teres and quadratus)
Wrist	Ulnar flexion	Flexor carpi ulnaris
Fingers	Flexion, ulnar deviation	Flexor digitorum (superficialis and profundus), lumbricales, interossei
Thumb	Flexion, adduction, opposition	Flexor pollicis (longus and brevis), adductor pollicis, opponens pollicis

Grip

Distal Hand

Your left hand contacts the palmar surface of the patient's hand. Your fingers are on the radial side (2nd metacarpal), your thumb gives counter-pressure on the ulnar border (5th metacarpal). There is no contact on the dorsal surface.

> **!** Caution: Do not squeeze the patient's hand.

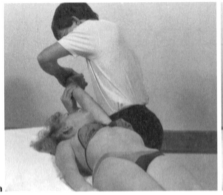 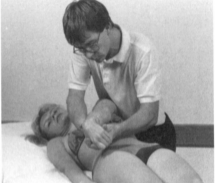

a   b

Fig. 7.5 a, b. Extension–adduction–internal rotation

Proximal Hand

Your right hand comes from the radial side and holds the patient's forearm just proximal to the wrist. Your fingers contact the ulnar border. Your thumb is on the radial border.

Elongated Position

Place the wrist in radial extension and the forearm into supination. Maintain the wrist and hand in position while you move the shoulder into flexion and abduction. You may use gentle traction to help elongate the shoulder and scapula muscles. The palm faces about 45° to the lateral plane. The traction brings the scapula into posterior elevation. Continuation of the traction elongates the patient's trunk diagonally from left to right. Too much abduction prevents trunk elongation. Too much external rotation prevents the scapula from coming into full posterior elevation.

If the patient has just completed the antagonistic motion (flexion–abduction–external rotation), begin at the end of that pattern.

Body Mechanics

Stand in a stride position above the patient's shoulder with your left foot forward. Face the line of motion. Start with the weight on your back foot and let the patient's motion pull your weight to your front foot. Continue facing the line of motion.

Stretch

Apply the stretch to the shoulder and hand simultaneously. Your proximal hand does a rapid traction with rotation of the shoulder and scapula.

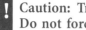 Caution: Do not force the shoulder into more flexion.

Your distal hand gives traction to the wrist.

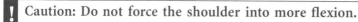 Caution: Traction the wrist in line with the metacarpal bones. Do not force the wrist into more extension.

Command

"Squeeze my hand, pull down and across." "Squeeze and pull!"

Movement

The fingers and thumb flex as the wrist moves into ulnar flexion. The radial side of the hand leads as the shoulder moves into extension with adduction and internal rotation and the scapula into anterior depression. Continuation of this motion brings the patient into trunk flexion with neck flexion to the right.

Resistance

Your distal hand combines traction through the flexed wrist with rotary resistance to ulnar deviation. The rotary resistance at the wrist provides resistance to the forearm pronation and shoulder adduction and internal rotation. The traction at the wrist resists the wrist flexion and the shoulder extension.

Your proximal hand combines a traction force with rotary resistance. The line of resistance is back toward the starting position. Maintaining the traction force will guide your resistance in the proper arc.

Your hands change from traction to approximation as the shoulder and scapula near the end of their range. The approximation resists the scapula depression and stabilizes the shoulder.

End Position

The scapula is in anterior depression. The shoulder is in extension, adduction, and internal rotation with the humerus crossing the midline to the right. The forearm is pronated, the wrist and fingers flexed with the palm facing toward the right ilium.

Timing for Emphasis

You may prevent motion in the beginning range of shoulder extension or allow the shoulder to reach the mid-position and exercise the wrist, hand, and fingers. To exercise the fingers and thumb, move your proximal hand to give resistance just distal to the wrist. Your distal hand can now exercise the fingers, together or individually.

→ **Points to remember**
- **The stretch at the wrist and shoulder is done with traction, not more flexion**
- **Approximate at the end range to resist the scapula and stabilize the shoulder**
- **The humerus crosses mid-line**

7.3.1 Extension–Adduction–Internal Rotation with Elbow Extension (Fig. 7.6)

Joint	Movement	Muscles: principal components (Kendall and McCreary 1983)
Scapula	Anterior depression	Serratus anterior (lower), pectoralis minor, rhomboids
Shoulder	Extension, Adduction, Internal Rotation	Pectoralis major, teres major, subscapularis
Elbow	Extension	Triceps, anconeus
Forearm	Pronation	Brachioradialis, pronator (teres and quadratus)
Wrist	Ulnar flexion	Flexor carpi ulnaris
Fingers	Flexion, ulnar deviation	Flexor digitorum (superficialis and profundus), lumbricales, interossei
Thumb	Flexion, adduction, opposition	Flexor pollicis (longus and brevis), adductor pollicis, opponens pollicis

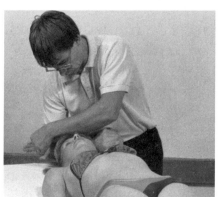

a

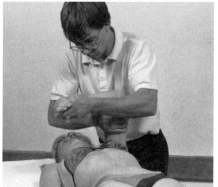

b

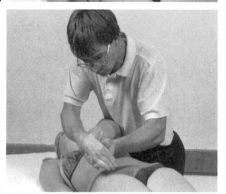

c

Fig. 7.6 a–c. Extension–adduction–internal rotation with elbow extension

Grip

Your distal grip is the same as for the straight arm pattern. Wrap your proximal hand around the humerus from underneath so that your fingers can give pressure opposite the direction of rotation. During the starting position the therapist can give resistance with the forearm against the forearm of the patient on the palmar side (Fig 7.6 a).

Elongated Position

The humerus is in full flexion with the scapula in posterior elevation. The elbow is flexed, and the patient's forearm is touching the head. The wrist is in full radial extension with the fingers extended.

Body Mechanics

Your body mechanics are the same as for the straight arm pattern.

Stretch

Apply the stretch to the shoulder and hand simultaneously. Your proximal hand does a rapid traction with rotation of the shoulder and scapula. Your distal hand gives traction to the wrist. Usually the patient's forearm is touching the head, preventing increased elbow flexion.

Command

"Squeeze my hand, push down and across, straighten your elbow." "Squeeze and push!" "Reach for your right hip."

Movement

The fingers and thumb flex and the wrist moves into ulnar flexion. The shoulder begins its motion into extension–adduction, and then the elbow begins to extend. The hand moves down toward the opposite hip. The elbow reaches full extension as the shoulder and scapula complete their motion.

Resistance

Your distal hand resists the wrist and forearm, as in the straight arm pattern. Give resistance to the elbow extension by rotating the forearm and hand back toward the starting position of elbow flexion. Give approximation to facilitate the elbow extension.

Your proximal hand gives traction through the humerus combined with rotary resistance back toward the starting position. Change from traction to approximation as the shoulder and scapula pass about halfway through their range.

Each of your hands uses the proper force to make the resistance appropriate for the strength of the elbow and the strength of the shoulder.

End Position

The end position is the same as the straight arm pattern.

Timing for Emphasis

Prevent elbow extension at the beginning of the range and exercise the shoulder. Lock in shoulder extension in mid-range and exercise the elbow extension with pronation.

→ **Points to remember**
- **The humerus crosses mid-line**
- **Normal timing: the elbow and shoulder motion occur together**

7.3.2 Extension–Adduction–Internal Rotation with Elbow Flexion (Fig. 7.7)

Joint	Movement	Muscles: principal components (Kendall and McCreary 1983)
Scapula	Anterior depression	Serratus anterior (lower), pectoralis minor, rhomboids
Shoulder	Extension, Adduction, Internal Rotation	Pectoralis major, teres major, subscapularis
Elbow	Flexion	Biceps, brachialis
Forearm	Pronation	Brachioradialis, pronator (teres and quadratus)
Wrist	Ulnar flexion	Flexor carpi ulnaris
Fingers	Flexion, ulnar deviation	Flexor digitorum (superficialis and profundus), lumbricales, interossei
Thumb	Flexion, adduction, opposition	Flexor pollicis (longus and brevis), adductor pollicis, opponens pollicis

Grip

Your distal and proximal grips are the same as those used for extension–adduction–internal rotation with elbow extension.

Alternative Grip

After the motion begins, the proximal hand may move to the scapula to emphasize that motion.

Elongated Position

The position is the same as the straight arm pattern.

Stretch

The stretch is the same as for the straight arm pattern.

Command

"Squeeze my hand, pull down and across and bend your elbow." "Squeeze and pull."

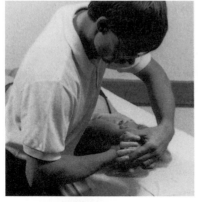

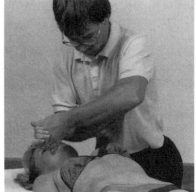

a

b

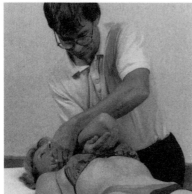

Fig. 7.7 a–e. Extension–adduction–internal rotation with elbow flexion. **a–c** Standard grips; **d,e** grip variations

c

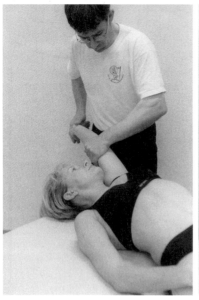

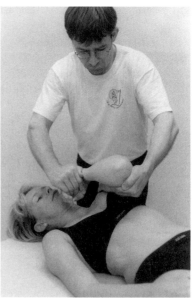

d

e

Movement

The fingers and thumb flex and the wrist moves into ulnar flexion. The shoulder starts into extension–adduction and the elbow begins to flex. The elbow reaches full flexion as the shoulder and scapula complete their motion.

Resistance

Your distal hand resists the wrist and forearm, as in the straight arm pattern. Give resistance to the elbow flexion by rotating the forearm toward supination and back toward the starting position of elbow extension.

Your proximal hand gives traction through the humerus combined with rotary resistance back toward the starting position. Change from traction to approximation as the shoulder and scapula pass about halfway through their range.

Each of your hands uses the proper force to make the resistance appropriate for the strength of the elbow and the strength of the shoulder.

End Position

The humerus is in extension with adduction, the scapula in anterior depression. The elbow is fully flexed. The wrist is in ulnar flexion and the hand closed. The rotation in the shoulder and forearm is the same as in the straight arm pattern. If you extend the patient's elbow, the position is the same as the straight arm pattern.

Timing for Emphasis

With the three moving segments, shoulder, elbow and wrist, you may again lock in any two and exercise the third.

With the elbow bent it is easy to exercise the internal rotation separately from the other motions. Exercise this motion where the strength of shoulder extension is greatest. You may work through the full range of shoulder internal rotation during these exercises and return to the groove before finishing the pattern.

When exercising the patient's wrist or hand, move your proximal hand to the forearm and give resistance to the shoulder and elbow by pulling back toward the starting position. Your distal hand is now free to give appropriate resistance to the wrist and hand. To exercise the fingers and thumb, move your proximal stabilizing hand just distal to the wrist.

You may prevent motion in the beginning range of shoulder extension and exercise the elbow, wrist, hand, or fingers. In addition, you may lock in the shoulder and elbow motion in mid-range to exercise the wrist and hand. This places the hand where the patient can see it as it moves.

→ **Points to remember**
- **With the proper rotation the humerus will cross mid-line**
- **Resist the elbow flexion with traction back toward the starting position**
- **Normal timing: the elbow and shoulder motion occur together**

7.4 Flexion–Adduction–External Rotation (Fig. 7.8)

Joint	Movement	Muscles: principal components (Kendall and McCreary 1983)
Scapula	Anterior elevation	Serratus anterior (upper), trapezius
Shoulder	Flexion, adduction, external rotation	Pectoralis major (upper) deltoid (anterior), biceps, coracobrachialis
Elbow	Extended (position unchanged)	Triceps, anconeus
Forearm	Supination	Brachioradialis, supinator
Wrist	Radial flexion	Flexor carpi radialis
Fingers	Flexion, radial deviation	Flexor digitorum (superficialis and profundus), lumbricales, interossei
Thumb	Flexion, adduction opposition	Flexor pollicis (longus and brevis), adductor pollicis, opponens pollicis

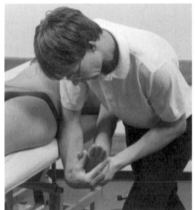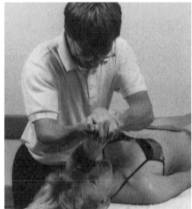

a   b

Fig. 7.8 a, b. Flexion–adduction–external rotation

Grip

Distal Hand

Your right hand contacts the palmar surface of the patient's hand. Your fingers are on the ulnar side (5th metacarpal), your thumb gives counter pressure on the radial side (2nd metacarpal). There is no contact on the dorsal surface.

> **!** Caution: Do not squeeze the hand.

Proximal Hand

Your left hand grips the patient's forearm from underneath just proximal to the wrist. Your fingers are on the radial side, your thumb on the ulnar side.

Alternative Grip

To emphasize shoulder or scapula motions, move the proximal hand to grip the upper arm or the scapula after the shoulder begins its motion.

Elongated Position

Place the wrist in ulnar extension and the forearm into pronation. Maintain the wrist and hand in position while you move the shoulder into extension and abduction. The palm faces about 45° in toward the body. The traction brings the scapula into posterior depression. Continuation of the traction shortens the left side of the patient's trunk. Too much shoulder abduction prevents the trunk motion and pulls the scapula out of position. Too much internal rotation tilts the scapula forward.

Body Mechanics

Stand in a stride position by the patient's elbow, facing toward the patient's feet. The patient's motion of flexion with external rotation pivots you around so you face diagonally up toward the patient's head. Let the patient's motion pull your weight from your back to your front foot.

Stretch

Your proximal hand does a rapid traction with rotation of the shoulder and scapula. At the same time your distal hand gives traction to the wrist.

> **!** Caution: Traction the wrist in line with the metacarpal bones. Do not force the wrist into more extension.

Command

"Squeeze my hand, pull up and across your nose." "Squeeze and pull."

Movement

The fingers and thumb flex as the wrist moves into radial flexion. The radial side of the hand leads as the shoulder moves into flexion with adduction and external rotation and the scapula into anterior elevation. Continuation of this motion elongates the patient's trunk with rotation toward the right.

Resistance

Your distal hand combines traction through the flexed wrist with rotary resistance to radial deviation. The rotary resistance at the wrist provides resistance to the forearm supination and to the shoulder adduction and external rotation. The traction force resists both the wrist flexion and shoulder flexion. At the end of the movement you may need to give approximation with the distal hand to stabilize the elbow in extension.

Your proximal hand combines a traction force with rotary resistance. The line of resistance is back toward the starting position. Maintaining the traction force guides your resistance in the proper arc.

Use approximation at the end of the motion to resist the scapula elevation and stabilize the shoulder and elbow.

End Position

The scapula is in anterior elevation, and the shoulder is in flexion and adduction with external rotation, the humerus crosses the midline (over the patient's face). The forearm is supinated, the elbow straight, and the wrist and fingers flexed. Continuation of the motion will cause the patient's trunk to rotate and extend to the right.

Timing for Emphasis

You may prevent motion in the beginning range of shoulder flexion or allow the shoulder to reach the mid-position and exercise the wrist, hand, or fingers. Lock in the forearm rotation or allow it to move with the wrist.

→ **Points to remember**
- The stretch at the wrist and shoulder is done with traction, not more extension
- Approximate with the distal hand to stabilize the elbow in extension at end range
- The humerus crosses mid-line (the nose when the patient's head is not turned)

7.4.1 Flexion–Adduction–External Rotation
with Elbow Flexion (Fig. 7.9)

Joint	Movement	Muscles: principal components (Kendall and McCreary 1983)
Scapula	Anterior elevation	Serratus anterior (upper), trapezius
Shoulder	Flexion, adduction, external rotation	Pectoralis major (upper) deltoid (anterior), biceps, coracobrachialis
Elbow	Flexion	Biceps, brachialis
Forearm	Supination	Brachioradialis, supinator
Wrist	Radial flexion	Flexor carpi radialis
Fingers	Flexion, radial deviation	Flexor digitorum (superficialis and profundus), lumbricales, interossei
Thumb	Flexion, adduction	Flexor pollicis (longus and brevis), adductor pollicis

Grip

Your distal grip is the same as used for the straight arm pattern. Your proximal hand may start with the grip for the straight arm pattern. As the shoulder and elbow begin to flex, move this hand up to grip the humerus. Wrap your hand around the humerus from the medial side and use your fingers to give pressure opposite the direction of motion. The resistance to rotation comes from the line of your fingers and forearm (Fig. 7.9).

Alternative Grip

The proximal hand may move to the scapula to emphasize that motion.

Elongated Position

Position the limb as for the straight arm pattern.

Body Mechanics

Your body mechanics are the same as for the straight arm pattern. Use your body weight for resistance.

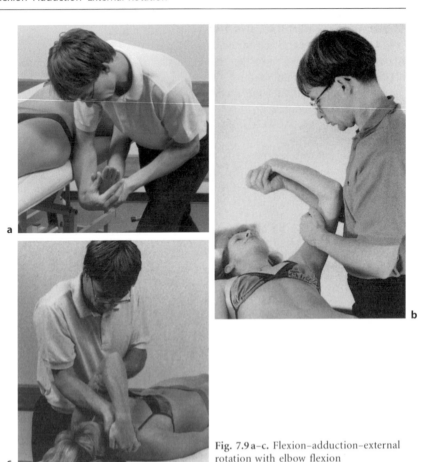

Fig. 7.9 a–c. Flexion–adduction–external rotation with elbow flexion

Stretch

Use the same motions for the stretch reflex that you used with the straight arm pattern.

> **!** Caution: Traction the wrist in line with the metacarpal bones. Do not force the wrist into more extension.

Command

"Squeeze my hand, pull up across your nose and bend your elbow." "Squeeze and pull." "Touch your right ear."

Movement

After the wrist flexes and the forearm supinates, the shoulder and elbow begin to flex. The shoulder and elbow move at the same speed and complete their movements at the same time.

Resistance

Your distal hand resists the wrist and forearm as in the straight arm pattern. That rotary resistance plus the traction back toward the starting position gives the resistance to elbow flexion. Your proximal hand rotates and gives traction to the humerus back toward the starting position.

Give a separate force with each hand so that the resistance is appropriate for the strength of the shoulder and elbow.

End Position

The patient's shoulder, forearm, and hand are positioned as in the straight arm pattern. The elbow is flexed, and the patient's fist may touch the right ear. The rotation in the shoulder and forearm are the same as in the straight arm pattern. Extend the elbow to check the amount of rotation.

Timing for Emphasis

With three moving segments, shoulder, elbow and wrist, you may lock in any two and exercise the third.

With the elbow bent it is easy to exercise the external rotation separately from the forearm rotation and the supination separately from the shoulder rotation. Do this where the strength of the shoulder and elbow flexion is greatest. If you work through the full range of shoulder external rotation, return to the groove before finishing the pattern.

You may lock in the shoulder flexion in mid-range and exercise the wrist, and the finger motions. In this position the patient can see the movements. When exercising the wrist or hand, move your proximal hand to the forearm or hand to stabilize and resist the proximal joints. Your other hand grips distal to the joints being exercised.

→ **Points to remember**
- **The humerus must cross mid-line, (the nose when the patient's head is not turned)**
- **Resistance to supination facilitates the elbow motion**

7.4.2 Flexion–Adduction–External Rotation with Elbow Extension (Fig. 7.10)

Joint	Movement	Muscles: principal components (Kendall and McCreary 1983)
Scapula	Anterior elevation	Serratus anterior (upper), trapezius
Shoulder	Flexion, adduction, external rotation	Pectoralis major (upper) deltoid (anterior), biceps, coracobrachialis
Elbow	Extension	Triceps, anconeus
Forearm	Supination	Brachioradialis, supinator
Wrist	Radial flexion	Flexor carpi radialis
Fingers	Flexion, radial deviation	Flexor digitorum (superficialis and profundus), lumbricales, interossei
Thumb	Flexion, adduction	Flexor pollicis (longus and brevis), adductor pollicis

Grip

Distal Hand

The distal grip is the same as used for the straight arm pattern.

Proximal Hand

Your proximal hand starts with the grip on the forearm used with the straight arm pattern. As the shoulder begins to flex and the elbow to extend, you can move your distal hand up to grip the humerus. Wrap your hand around the humerus from the medial side and use your fingers to give pressure opposite the direction of motion. You may use the grip on the humerus from the start of the pattern.

Elongated Position

Start by positioning the limb as you did for the straight arm pattern. Maintain traction on the shoulder and scapula with your proximal hand while you use that hand to flex the elbow. Your distal hand tractions the wrist into ulnar extension. If you begin with your left hand on the humerus, your distal (right) hand flexes the elbow.

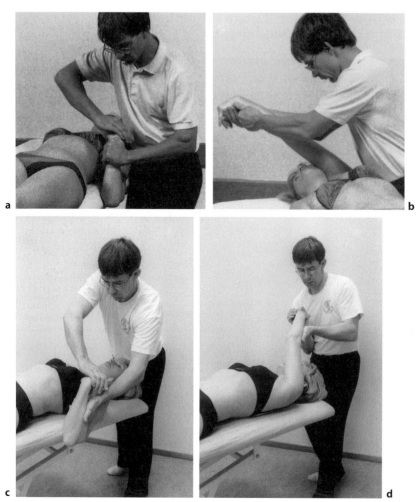

Fig. 7.10a–d. Flexion–adduction–external rotation with elbow extension. **a,b** The therapist is standing on the same side of the table; **c,d** the therapist is standing on the other side of the table

Body Mechanics

Your body mechanics are the same as for the straight arm pattern. Use your body weight for resistance.

Stretch

Your proximal hand does a rapid traction with rotation of the shoulder and scapula. At the same time your distal hand gives traction to the wrist.

> ❗ Caution: Do not force the wrist into more extension.

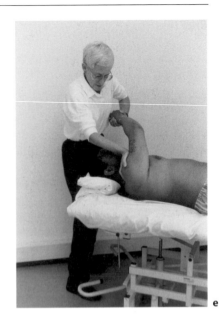

Fig. 7.10 e. Flexion–adduction–external rotation with elbow extension. Patient with right hemiplegia: the therapist's proximal hand facilitates scapula anterior elevation and trunk elongation

e

Command

"Squeeze my hand, push up and across your nose and straighten your elbow." "Squeeze and push!" "Reach up across your nose."

Movement

First the wrist flexes and the forearm supinates. Then the shoulder begins to flex and elbow to extend. The shoulder and elbow should complete their motions at the same time.

Resistance

Your distal hand resists the wrist and forearm as in the straight arm pattern. Added is the rotary resistance to elbow extension.

Your proximal hand rotates and tractions the humerus back toward the starting position.

Give a separate force with each hand so that the resistance is appropriate for the strength of the shoulder and elbow. Give approximation at the end range to stabilize the elbow, shoulder and scapula.

End Position

The patient's shoulder, forearm, and hand are positioned as in the straight arm pattern.

Timing for Emphasis

The emphasis here is to teach the patient to combine shoulder flexion with elbow extension in a smooth motion.

Alternative Grip and Body Mechanics

The therapist can also stand on the head side of the table in the line of the motion. The distal grip is the same and the proximal grip is on the forearm on the flexor muscle group (Fig. 7.10 c–e).

→ **Points to remember**
- **Resistance to the elbow extension is rotary and back toward the starting position**
- **Normal timing: the elbow and shoulder motion occur together**

7.5 **Extension–Abduction–Internal Rotation** (Fig. 7.11)

Joint	Movement	Muscles: principal components (Kendall and McCreary 1983)
Scapula	Posterior depression	Rhomboids
Shoulder	Extension, Abduction, Internal Rotation	Latissimus dorsi, deltoid (middle, posterior), triceps, teres major, subscapularis
Elbow	Extended (position unchanged)	Triceps, anconeus
Forearm	Pronation	Brachioradialis, pronator (teres and quadratus)
Wrist	Ulnar extension	Extensor carpi ulnaris
Fingers	Extension, ulnar deviation	Extensor digitorum longus, lumbricales, interossei
Thumb	Palmar abduction, extension	Abductor pollicis (brevis), Extensor pollicis

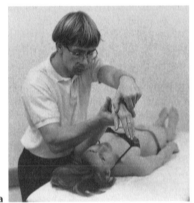

a

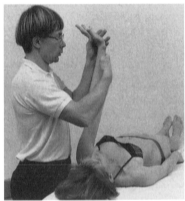

b

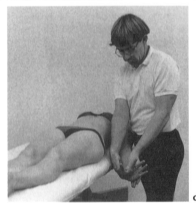

c

Fig. 7.11 a–c. Extension–abduction–internal rotation

Grip

Distal Hand

Your left hand grips the dorsal surface of the patient's hand. Your fingers are on the ulnar side (5th metacarpal), your thumb gives counter-pressure on the radial side (2nd metacarpal). There is no contact on the palm.

 Caution: Do not squeeze the hand.

Proximal Hand

With your hand facing the ventral surface, use the lumbrical grip to hold the radial and ulnar sides of the patient's forearm proximal to the wrist.

Alternative Grip

To emphasize shoulder or scapula motions, move the proximal hand to the upper arm or to the scapula after the shoulder begins to extend.

Elongated Position

Place the wrist in radial flexion and the forearm into supination. Maintain the wrist and hand in position while you move the shoulder into flexion and adduction. Use gentle traction to bring the scapula into anterior elevation and help elongate the shoulder muscles. The humerus crosses over the patient's nose and the palm faces toward the patient's right ear. A continuation of this motion would bring the patient into trunk elongation with rotation to the right.

If the patient has just completed the antagonistic motion (flexion–adduction–external rotation), begin at the end of that pattern.

Body Mechanics

Stand in a stride position in the line of the motion facing toward the patient's hand. Start with the weight on your front foot and let the patient's motion push your weight to your back foot. Move your trunk to the right to allow the arm motion and to control the pronation with your distal grip. As the patient's arm nears the end of the range, your body turns so you face the patient's feet.

Stretch

Apply the stretch to the shoulder and hand simultaneously. Your proximal hand does a rapid traction with rotation of the shoulder and scapula. Combine this motion with traction to the wrist with your distal hand.

 Caution: Traction the wrist in line with the metacarpal bones. Do not force the wrist into more flexion.

Command

"Hand back, push your arm down to your side." "Push!"

Movement

The fingers and thumb extend as the wrist moves into ulnar extension. The ulnar side of the hand leads as the shoulder moves into extension with abduction and internal rotation. The scapula moves into posterior depression. Continuation of this motion is a downward reach toward the back of the left heel with shortening of the left side of the trunk.

Resistance

Your distal hand combines traction through the extended wrist with a rotary resistance for the ulnar deviation. The resistance to the forearm pronation and the shoulder internal rotation and abduction comes from the rotary resistance at the wrist. The traction force resists the motions of wrist and shoulder extension.

Your proximal hand combines a traction force with rotary resistance. The line of resistance is back toward the starting position.

As the patient's arm nears the end of the range of extension, both hands change from a traction to an approximation force.

End Position

The scapula is in full posterior depression. The humerus is in extension at the left side, the forearm is pronated, and the palm is facing about 45° to the lateral plane. The wrist is in ulnar extension, the fingers are extended toward the ulnar side, and the thumb is extended and abducted at right angles to the palm.

Timing for Emphasis

You may prevent motion in the beginning of the shoulder extension and exercise the wrist, hand, or fingers. This position puts the hand where the patient can see it during the exercise.

> → **Points to remember**
> - Let the patient's motion do the work of pushing your weight to your back foot
> - At the end of the range both hands change their force from traction to approximation

7.5.1 Extension–Abduction–Internal Rotation with Elbow Extension (Fig. 7.12)

Joint	Movement	Muscles: principal components (Kendall and McCreary 1983)
Scapula	Posterior depression	Rhomboids
Shoulder	Extension, Abduction, Internal Rotation	Latissimus dorsi, deltoid (middle, posterior), triceps, teres major, subscapularis
Elbow	Extension	Triceps, anconeus
Forearm	Pronation	Brachioradialis, pronator (teres and quadratus)
Wrist	Ulnar extension	Extensor carpi ulnaris
Fingers	Extension, ulnar deviation	Extensor digitorum longus, lumbricales, interossei
Thumb	Palmar abduction, extension	Abductor pollicis (brevis), Extensor pollicis

Grip

Distal Hand

Your distal grip is the same as used for the straight arm pattern.

Proximal Hand

Wrap your hand around the humerus so your fingers can give pressure opposite the direction of internal rotation.

Alternative Grip

The proximal hand may move to the scapula to emphasize the posterior depression.

Elongated Position

The position of the scapula, shoulder, forearm, and wrist are the same as for the straight arm pattern. The patient's elbow is fully flexed.

Body Mechanics

Your body mechanics are the same as for the straight arm pattern.

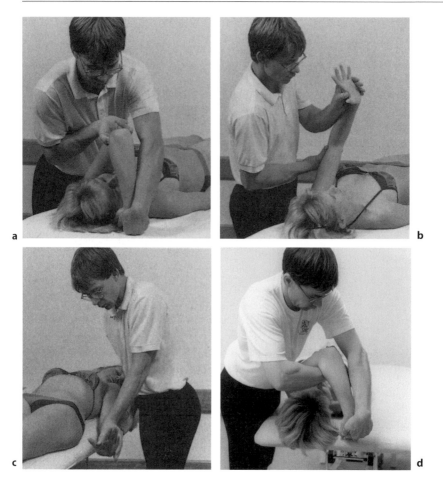

Fig. 7.12a–d. Extension–abduction–internal rotation with elbow extension. **d** Different proximal grip

Stretch

Apply the stretch to the shoulder, elbow, and hand simultaneously. The stretch of the shoulder comes from a rapid traction with rotation of the shoulder and scapula by the proximal hand. The distal hand continues giving traction to the hand and wrist while increasing the elbow supination. Stretch the elbow into more flexion if there is space.

> **!** Caution: Traction the wrist; do not force it into more flexion.

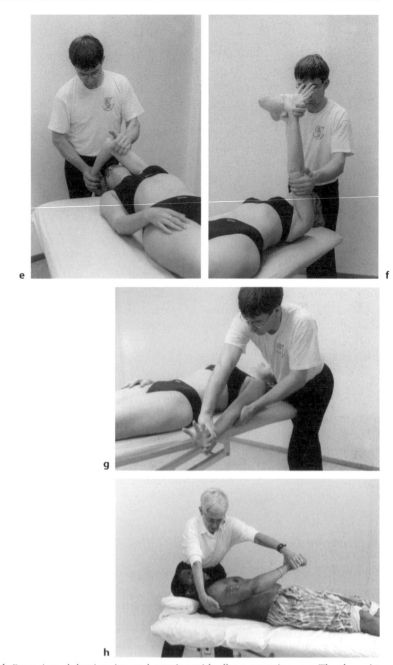

Fig. 7.12 e–h Extension–abduction–internal rotation with elbow extension. e–g The therapist on the opposite side of the table. h Patient with right hemiplegia: the therapist facilitates the scapula and trunk with her proximal hand

Command

"Hand up, push your arm down toward me and straighten your elbow as you go." "Push!"

Movement

The fingers extend and the wrist moves into ulnar extension. The shoulder begins its motion into extension–abduction, and then the elbow begins to extend. The elbow reaches full extension as the shoulder and scapula complete their motion.

Resistance

Your distal hand resists the wrist and forearm as in the straight arm pattern. Give resistance to the elbow extension by rotating the forearm and hand back toward the starting position of elbow flexion.

Your proximal hand gives traction through the humerus combined with rotary resistance back toward the starting position. When the shoulder and elbow near full extension, change from traction to approximation.

End Position

The end position is the same as the straight arm pattern.

Timing for Emphasis

Prevent elbow extension at the beginning of the range and exercise the shoulder. Prevent shoulder extension at the beginning of the range and exercise the elbow extension with pronation. Lock in the shoulder extension in mid-range and exercise both the elbow extension with pronation and the wrist ulnar extension.

Alternative Grip and Body Mechanics

The therapist can also stand at the head of the table on the opposite side. The distal grip is the same. Grip with your proximal hand around the posterior surface of the humerus from the lateral side. Face the diagonal and use your body weight for resistance.

> → **Points to remember**
> - **Normal timing: the shoulder and elbow extend at the same rate**
> - **The rotational resistance with your distal hand facilitates the elbow and wrist extension**

7.5.2 Extension–Abduction–Internal Rotation with Elbow Flexion (Fig. 7.13)

Joint	Movement	Muscles: principal components (Kendall and McCreary 1983)
Scapula	Posterior depression	Rhomboids
Shoulder	Extension, Abduction, Internal Rotation	Latissimus dorsi, deltoid (middle, posterior), triceps, teres major, subscapularis
Elbow	Flexion	Biceps, brachialis
Forearm	Pronation	Brachioradialis, pronator (teres and quadratus)
Wrist	Ulnar extension	Extensor carpi ulnaris
Fingers	Extension, ulnar deviation	Extensor digitorum longus, lumbricales, interossei
Thumb	Palmar abduction, extension	Abductor pollicis (brevis), Extensor pollicis

Grip

Distal Hand

Your distal grip is the same as used for the straight arm pattern.

Proximal Hand

Your proximal hand may start with the grip on the forearm. As the shoulder and elbow motions begin, wrap your proximal hand around the humerus from underneath. Your fingers give pressure opposite the direction of rotation and resist the shoulder extension.

Alternative Grip

You may also move your proximal hand to the scapula to emphasize that motion.

Body Mechanics

These are the same as for the straight arm pattern.

Alternative Grip and Body Mechanics

You may stand on the opposite side of the table. Face the diagonal and use your body weight for resistance (Fig. 7.14).

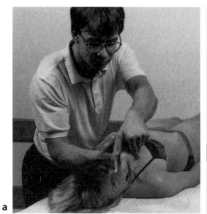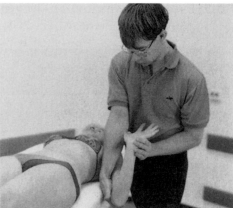

a   b

Fig. 7.13. Extension–abduction–internal rotation with elbow flexion

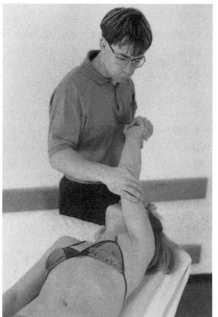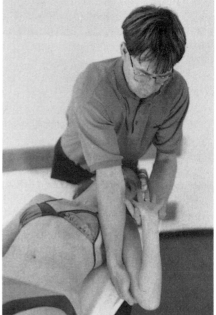

a   b

Fig. 7.14a,b. Extension–abduction–internal rotation with elbow flexion: therapist at the head end of the table

Elongated Position

The position is the same as for the straight arm pattern.

Stretch

The stretch is the same as for the straight arm pattern.

Command

"Fingers and wrist back, push down and out and bend your elbow." "Push down and bend your elbow." If you are standing on the opposite side of the table the command is "Pull down."

Movement

The fingers extend and the wrist moves into ulnar extension. The shoulder begins its motion into extension–abduction, then the elbow begins to flex. The elbow reaches full flexion as the shoulder and scapula complete their motion.

Resistance

The distal hand gives the same resistance to the shoulder movement as in the straight arm pattern and a flexion resistance for the elbow.

At the start with the proximal hand on the forearm, it gives the same resistance as with the straight arm pattern. As soon as that hand moves to the upper arm, it gives resistance to rotation and shoulder extension. Change the traction on the humerus into approximation at the end of the movement.

End Position

The scapula is in posterior depression, the humerus in extension with abduction. The elbow is fully flexed. The wrist is again in ulnar extension and the hand open. The rotation in the shoulder and forearm are the same as in the straight arm pattern.

Timing for Emphasis

Lock in the wrist extension and elbow flexion, then exercise the shoulder in hyperextension and the scapula in posterior depression. When elbow flexion is stronger than extension, use this combination to exercise the patient's wrist and fingers.

→ **Points to remember**
- Normal timing: the shoulder and elbow complete their movements at the same time
- Extend the patient's elbow, the position is the same as the straight arm pattern.
- Change the traction on the humerus to approximation at the end of the movement

7.6 Thrust and Withdrawal Patterns

In the upper extremity patterns certain combinations of motions are fixed. The shoulder and forearm rotate in the same direction, supination occurs with external rotation and pronation with internal rotation. Extension of the hand and wrist is combined with shoulder abduction, flexion of the hand and wrist with shoulder adduction. The elbow is free to move in any direction or maintain its position.

The thrust combinations are associated with shoulder *adduction*. The fingers, the wrist and the elbow extend. The shoulder and forearm rotate in *opposite* directions from each other.

Thrust reversal (withdrawal) combinations are associated with shoulder *abduction*. The fingers, the wrist and the elbow flex. The shoulder and forearm rotate in *opposite directions* from each other.

Use these combinations when they are stronger than the normal pattern.

Example

Use ulnar withdrawal to strengthen shoulder extension and scapular posterior depression when elbow flexion with supination is stronger than elbow flexion or extension with pronation.

Example

Shoulder flexion–adduction with elbow extension is a good combination to facilitate rolling over from supine to prone. Use the ulnar thrust when elbow extension with pronation is more effective than forearm supination.

Therapist Position

The therapist's position remains in the line of the motion. Because of the "pushing" and "pulling" motions of the thrust-withdrawal diagonals, an effective position is at the opposite side of the patient. This position is illustrated with both thrust diagonals.

Grips

The distal and proximal grips are those used to resist the same distal and proximal pattern movements.

Timing

The sequencing of the movements is the same as it is in the patterns. The hand and wrist complete their motion, and then the elbow, shoulder and scapula move through their ranges together.

Timing for Emphasis

The thrust and withdrawal patterns are always exercised as a unit. Do the patterns singly or in combinations. Lock in the strong arm to reinforce the work of the weaker arm. Combination of Isotonics and Dynamic Reversals (Slow Reversals) work well with these patterns.

7.6.1 Ulnar Thrust and Withdrawal

Ulnar Thrust (Fig. 7.15)

The wrist and fingers extend with ulnar deviation and the elbow extends with forearm pronation. The shoulder moves into flexion–adduction–external rotation with scapular anterior elevation.

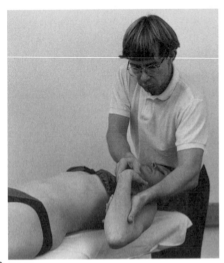 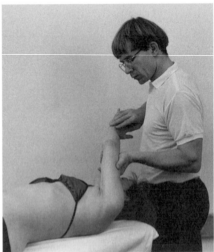

a b

Fig. 7.15 a, b. Ulnar thrust

Withdrawal from Ulnar Thrust (Fig. 7.16)

The wrist and fingers flex with radial deviation and the elbow flexes with forearm supination. The shoulder moves into extension–abduction–internal rotation with scapular posterior depression.

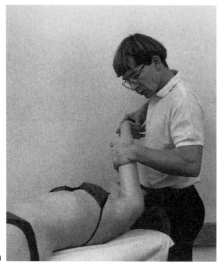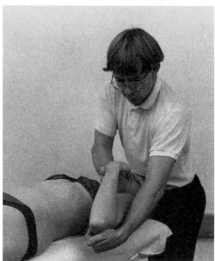

a   b

Fig. 7.16a,b. Withdrawal from ulnar thrust

7.6.2 Radial Thrust and Withdrawal

Radial Thrust (Fig. 7.17)

The wrist and fingers extend with radial deviation and the elbow extends with forearm supination. The shoulder moves into extension–adduction–internal rotation with scapular anterior depression.

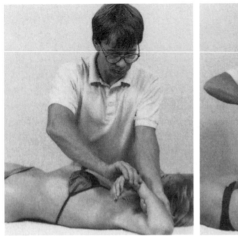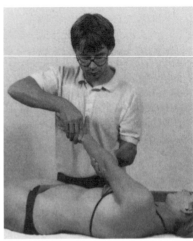

a   b

Fig. 7.17 a, b. Radial thrust

Withdrawal from Radial Thrust (Fig. 7.18)

The wrist and fingers flex with ulnar deviation and the elbow flexes with forearm pronation. The shoulder moves into flexion–abduction–external rotation with scapular posterior elevation.

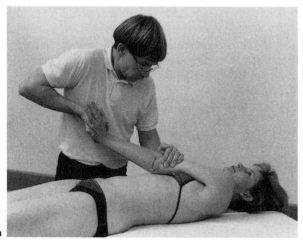

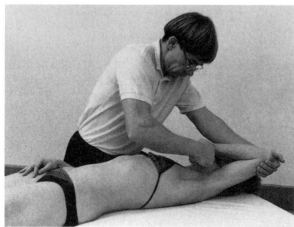

Fig. 7.18 a, b. Withdrawal from radial thrust

7.7 Bilateral Arm Patterns

Bilateral arm work allows you to use irradiation from the patient's strong arm to facilitate weak motions or muscles in the involved arm. You can use any combination of patterns in any position. Work with those that give you and the patient the greatest advantage in strength and control.

When you exercise both arms at the same time there is always more demand on the trunk muscles than when only one arm is exercising. You can increase this demand on the trunk by putting your patient in less supported positions such as sitting, kneeling, or standing. Bilateral combinations are very effective way to use the strong arm to reinforce the weaker arm.

Here we picture all the bilateral arm patterns with the patient supine to show the therapist's body position and grips more clearly.

Bilateral *Symmetrical.* Flexion–abduction–external rotation (Fig. 7.19).

Bilateral *Asymmetrical.* Flexion–abduction–external rotation with the right arm, flexion–adduction–external rotation with the left arm (Fig. 7.20).

Bilateral *Symmetrical Reciprocal.* Flexion–abduction–external rotation with the right arm, extension–adduction–internal rotation with the left arm (Fig. 7.21).

Bilateral *Asymmetrical Reciprocal.* Extension–adduction–internal rotation with the right arm, flexion–adduction–external rotation with the left arm (Fig. 7.22).

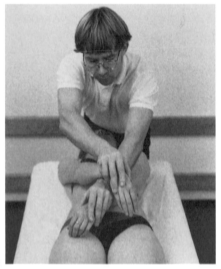 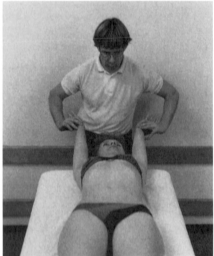

a   b

Fig. 7.19 a, b. Bilateral symmetrical patterns, flexion–abduction

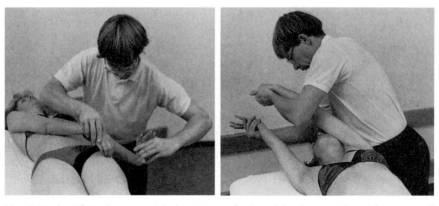

Fig. 7.20 a, b. Bilateral asymmetrical patterns, flexion–abduction on the right arm and flexion–adduction on the left arm

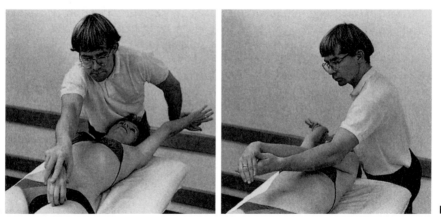

Fig. 7.21 a, b. Bilateral symmetrical reciprocal patterns, flexion–abduction on the right arm and extension–adduction on the left arm

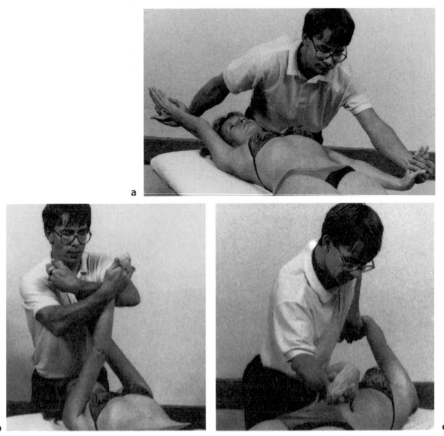

Fig. 7.22 a–c. Bilateral asymmetrical reciprocal patterns, extension–adduction on the right arm and flexion–adduction on the left arm

7.8 Changing the Patient's Position

There are many advantages to exercising the patient's arms in a variety of positions. These include letting the patient see the arm, adding or eliminating the effect of gravity from a motion, and working with functional motions in functional positions. There are also disadvantages for each position. Choose the positions that give the desired benefits with the fewest drawbacks.

7.8.1 Arm Patterns in a Side Lying Position

In this position the patient is free to move and stabilize the scapula without interference from the supporting surface. You may stabilize the patient's trunk with external support or the patient may do the work of stabilizing the trunk.

Extension–abduction–internal rotation is shown in Fig. 7.23.

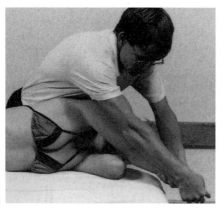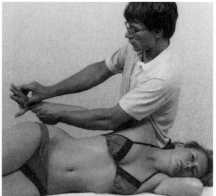

a   b

Fig. 7.23 a, b. Extension–abduction–internal rotation in the side lying position: **a** elongated position; **b** end position

7.8.2 Arm Patterns Lying Prone on Elbows

Working with the patient in this position allows you to exercise the end range of the shoulder abduction patterns against gravity. The scapula is free to move and stabilize without interference. The patient must bear weight on the other shoulder and scapula and maintain the head against gravity while exercising.

Flexion–abduction–external rotation at end range is shown in Fig. 7.24.

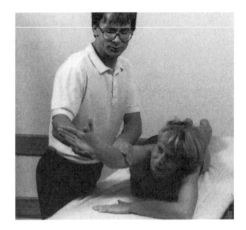

Fig. 7.24. Prone on elbows, arm pattern flexion–abduction–external rotation in the end position

7.8.3 Arm Patterns in a Sitting Position

In this position you can exercise the patient's arms through their full range or limit the work to functional motions such as eating, reaching, dressing. Bilateral arm patterns may be done to challenge the patient's balance and stability (Fig. 7.25).

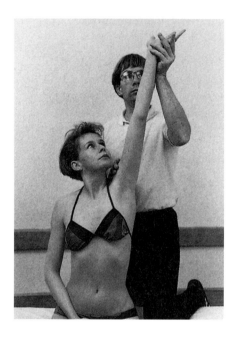

Fig. 7.25. Sitting position, arm pattern flexion–abduction–external rotation with visual reinforcement

7.8.4 Arm Patterns in the Quadruped Position

Working in this position, the patient must stabilize the trunk and bear weight on one arm while moving the other. As in the prone position, the shoulder muscles work against gravity (Fig. 7.26).

> **!** Caution: Do not allow the spine to move into undesired positions or postures.

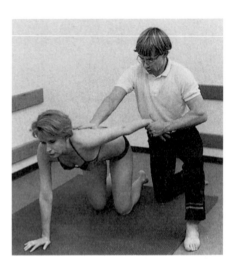

Fig. 7.26. Quadruped position, arm pattern extension–abduction–internal rotation

7.8.5 Arm Patterns in a Kneeling Position

Working in this position requires the patient to stabilize both the trunk, hips and knees while doing arm exercises (Fig. 7.27).

> **!** Caution: Do not allow the spine to move into undesired positions or postures.

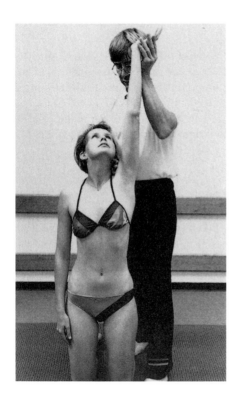

Fig. 7.27. Exercise in a kneeling position, irradiation from the arm pattern flexion–abduction–external rotation for extension of the trunk and hip

Reference

Kendal FP, McCreary EK (1983) Muscles, testing and function. Williams and Wilkins, Baltimore

8 The Lower Extremity

8.1 Introduction and Basic Procedures

Lower extremity patterns are used to treat dysfunctions in the pelvis, leg and foot caused by muscular weakness, incoordination, and joint restrictions. We can use these leg patterns for treatment of functional problems in walking and climbing up and down stairs, with activities such as rolling, and moving in bed. Your imagination can supply other examples. The leg patterns are also used to exercise the trunk. Resistance to strong leg muscles produces irradiation into weaker muscles elsewhere in the body.

We can use all the techniques with the leg patterns. The choice of individual techniques or combinations of techniques will depend on the patient's condition and the treatment goals. You can, for instance, combine Dynamic Reversals with Combination of Isotonics, Repeated Contractions with Dynamic Reversals or Contract-Relax or Hold-Relax with Combination of Isotonics and Dynamic Reversals.

Diagonal Motion

The lower extremity has two diagonals:
- Flexion–abduction–internal rotation and extension–adduction–external rotation
- Flexion–adduction–external rotation and extension–abduction–internal rotation

The hip and the ankle-foot complex are tied together in the pattern synergy. The knee is free to move into flexion, move into extension, or remain motionless. The leg moves through the diagonals in a straight line with the rotation occurring smoothly throughout the motion. In the normal timing of the pattern, the toes, foot and ankle move through their full range first, the other joints then move through their ranges together.

The basic patterns of the left leg with the subject supine are shown. All descriptions refer to this arrangement. To work with the right leg just change

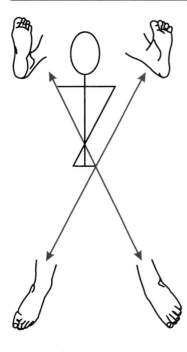

Fig. 8.1. Lower extremity diagonals (Courtesy of V. Jung)

the word "left" to "right" in the instructions. We can exercise leg patterns in different positions: prone, supine, side lying, quadruped, long sitting, side-sitting and in standing. Choose the position depending on the abilities of the patient, the treatment-goals, the influence of gravity, etc. Variations of position are shown later in the chapter.

Patient Position

! Note: Position the patient close to the edge of the table.

The patient's spine should be in a neutral position without side-bending or rotation. Before beginning a lower extremity pattern, visualize the patient's leg in a middle position where the lines of the two diagonals cross. Starting with the hip in neutral rotation, move the extremity into the elongated range of the pattern with the proper rotation, beginning with the foot and ankle.

Therapist Position

! Note: The therapist stands on the left side of the table with his or her pelvis facing the line of the diagonal, arms and hands aligned with the motion.

All grips described in the first part of each section assume that you are in this position. We first give the basic position and body mechanics for exercising the straight leg pattern. When we describe variations in the patterns we identify any changes in position or body mechanics. Some of these variations are pictured at the end of the chapter.

Grips

The grips follow the basic procedures for manual contact, that is, opposite the direction of movement. The first part of this chapter (Sect. 8.2) describes the two-handed grip used when the therapist stands next to the moving lower extremity. The basic grip is described for each straight leg pattern. The grips are modified when the therapist's or patient's position is changed. The grips also change when the therapist uses only one hand while the other hand controls a pattern on another extremity.

The grip on the foot contacts the active surface, dorsal or plantar, and holds the sides of the foot to resist the rotary components. Using the lumbrical grip will prevent squeezing or pinching the patient's foot. Remember, *pain inhibits effective motion.*

Resistance

The direction of the resistance is in an arc back toward the starting position. The angle of the therapist's hands and arms giving the resistance changes as the limb moves through the pattern.

Traction and Approximation

Traction and approximation are an important part of the resistance. Use traction at the beginning of the motion in both flexion and extension. Use approximation to stabilize the limb when it is in extension and traction to stabilize the limb in flexion.

Normal Timing and Timing for Emphasis

Normal Timing

The foot and ankle (distal component) begin the pattern by moving through their full range. Rotation at the hip and knee accompanies the rotation (eversion or inversion) of the foot. After the distal movement is completed, the hip or hip and knee move jointly through their range.

Timing for Emphasis

In the sections on timing for emphasis we offer some suggestions for exercising components of the patterns. Any of the techniques may be used. We have found that Repeated Stretch (Repeated Contractions) and

Combination of Isotonics work well. Do not limit yourself to the exercises we suggest in this section, use your imagination.

Stretch

In the leg patterns we use stretch-stimulus with or without the stretch-reflex to facilitate an easier or stronger movement, or to start the motion. When stretching a pattern it is important to start with elongation of the distal component. Maintain the ankle and foot in its stretched position while you elongate the rest of the synergistic muscles.

Repeated Stretch (Repeated Contractions) during the motion facilitates a stronger motion or guides the motion into the desired direction. Repeated Stretch at the beginning of the pattern is used when the patient has difficulty initiating the motion and to guide the direction of the motion. To get the stretch-reflex the therapist must elongate both the distal and proximal components. Be sure you do not overstretch a muscle or put too much tension on joint structure. This is particularly important when the hip is extended with the knee flexed.

Irradiation and Reinforcement

We can use strong leg patterns (single or bilateral) to get irradiation into all other parts of our body. The patient's position in combination with the amount of resistance will control the amount of irradiation. We can use this irradiation to strengthen or mobilize other parts of our body, to relax muscle chains, or to facilitate a functional activity such as rolling.

8.2 **Flexion–Abduction–Internal Rotation** (Fig. 8.2)

Joint	Movement	Muscles: principal components (Kendall and McCreary 1983)
Hip	Flexion, abduction, internal rotation	Tensor fascia lata, rectus femoris, gluteus medius (anterior), gluteus minimus
Knee	Extended (position unchanged)	Quadriceps
Ankle/foot	Dorsiflexion, eversion	Peroneus tertius
Toes	Extension, lateral deviation	Extensor hallucis, extensor digitorum

Grip

Distal Hand

Your left hand grips the dorsum of the patient's foot. Your fingers are on the lateral border and your thumb gives counter-pressure on the medial border. Hold the sides of the foot but don't put any contact on the plantar surface. To avoid blocking toe motion, keep your grip proximal to the metatarsal-phalangeal joints. Do not squeeze or pinch the foot.

Proximal Hand

Place your right hand on the anterior-lateral surface of the thigh just proximal to the knee. The fingers are on the top, the thumb on the lateral surface.

Elongated Position

Traction the entire limb while you move the foot into plantar flexion and inversion. Continue the traction and maintain the external rotation as you place the hip into extension (touching the table) and adduction. Elongate the leg parallel to the table, don't push the leg into the table. The thigh crosses the midline, and the left side of the trunk elongates. If there is restriction in the range of hip adduction or external rotation the patient's pelvis will move toward the right. If the hip extension is restricted, the pelvis will move into anterior tilt.

Therapist's Position and Body Mechanics

Stand in a stride position by the patient's left hip with your right foot behind. Face toward the patient's foot and align your body with the line of motion of the pattern. Start with the weight on your front foot and let the motion of the patient's leg push you back over your right leg. If the patient's leg is long, you may have to step back with your left foot as your weight shifts farther back. Continue facing the line of motion.

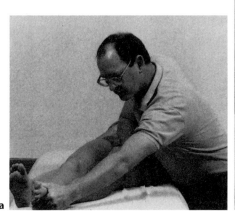
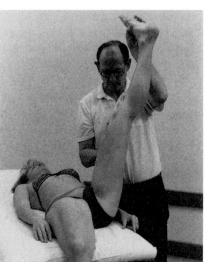

a   b

Fig. 8.2 a, b. Flexion–abduction–internal rotation

Alternative Position

You may stand on the right side of the table facing up toward the patient's left hip. If you choose this position, move the patient to the right side of the table. Your right hand is on the patient's foot, your left hand on the thigh. Stand in a stride with your right leg forward. As the patient's leg moves up into flexion, step forward with your left leg. This position makes it easier to get a good elongation at the beginning of the pattern. See Fig. 8.3 for an illustration of the alternative position.

Stretch

The reflex comes from a rapid elongation and rotation of the ankle, foot, and hip, by both hands simultaneously.

Command

"Foot up, lift your leg up and out." "Lift up!"

Movement

The toes extend as the foot and ankle move into dorsiflexion and eversion. The eversion promotes the hip internal rotation, and these motions occur almost simultaneously. The fifth metatarsal leads as the hip moves into flexion with abduction and internal rotation. Continuation of this motion produces trunk flexion with left side-bending.

Resistance

Your distal hand combines resistance to eversion with traction through the dorsiflexed foot. The resistance to the hip abduction and internal rotation comes from resisting eversion. The traction resists both the dorsiflexion and hip flexion. Your proximal hand combines traction through the line of the femur with a rotary force that resists the internal rotation and abduction. Maintaining the traction force will guide your resistance in the proper arc.

 Caution: Too much resistance to hip flexion may result in strain on the spine.

End Position

The foot is in dorsiflexion with eversion. The knee is in full extension and the hip in full flexion with enough abduction and internal rotation to align the knee and heel approximately with the lateral border of the left shoulder.

 Caution: The length of the hamstring muscles or other posterior structures may limit the hip motion. Do not allow the pelvis to move into a posterior tilt.

Timing for Emphasis

Prevent motion in the beginning range of hip flexion and exercise the foot and toes.

→ **Points to remember**
- **Start with good elongation of the leg, the thigh must start across mid-line**
- **Continuation of the elongation will lengthen the trunk lateral flexors**
- **The lumbar spine must remain in neutral**
- **Internal rotation of the hip is necessary, don't move only the foot**
- **Give traction to the femur during the motion**

8.2.1 Flexion–Abduction–Internal Rotation with Knee Flexion
(Fig. 8.3)

Joint	Movement	Muscles: principal components (Kendall and McCreary 1983)
Hip	Flexion, abduction, internal rotation	Tensor fascia lata, rectus femoris, gluteus medius (anterior), gluteus minimus
Knee	Flexion	Hamstrings, gracilis, gastrocnemius
Ankle/foot	Dorsiflexion, eversion	Peroneus tertius
Toes	Extension, lateral deviation	Extensor hallucis, extensor digitorum

Grip

Your distal and proximal grips remain the same as they were for the straight leg pattern.

Elongated Position

Position the limb as you did for the straight leg pattern.

Body Mechanics

Stand in the same stride position by the patient's hip as for the straight leg pattern. Again, allow the patient's motion to shift your weight from the front to the back foot. Face the line of motion.

Alternative Positions

You may use the same alternative position, standing on the opposite side of the table, as you used for the straight leg pattern (Fig. 8.3 c, d).

Stretch

Use the same motions for the stretch that you used with the straight leg pattern. Traction with the distal hand will facilitate the knee flexors.

Command

"Foot up, bend your knee up and out." "Bend up!"

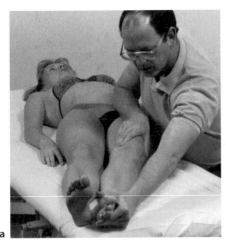
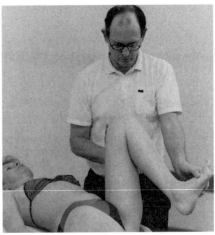

a

b

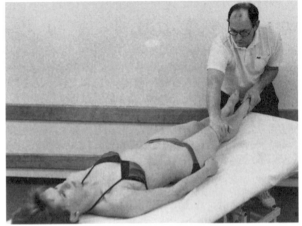

c

Fig. 8.3 a–d. Flexion–
abduction–internal
rotation with knee
flexion. a, b Usual
position of the therapist;
c, d alternative position
on the opposite side of
the table

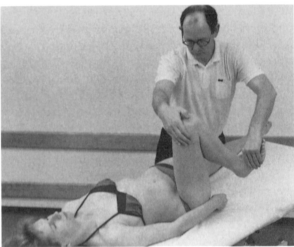

d

Movement

The foot and ankle dorsiflex and evert. The hip and knee motions begin next and both joints reach their end ranges at the same time. Continuation of this motion also causes trunk flexion with lateral flexion to the left.

Resistance

Give traction with your proximal hand through the line of the femur, adding a rotary force, to resist the hip motion. Resist the foot and ankle motion as before with your distal hand. Resist the knee flexion by applying traction through the tibia toward the starting position. The resistance to knee flexion is crucial to successful use of this combination for strengthening the hip and trunk.

End Position

The foot is in dorsiflexion with eversion. The hip and knee are in full flexion with the heel close to the lateral border of the buttock. The knee and heel are aligned with each other and lined up approximately with the lateral border of the left shoulder.

Note: If you extend the patient's knee the position is the same as the straight leg pattern.

Timing for Emphasis

With three moving segments, hip, knee, and foot, you may lock in any two and exercise the third. With the knee bent it is easy to exercise the internal rotation separately from the other hip motions. Do these exercises where the strength of the hip flexion is greatest. You may work through the full range of hip internal rotation during these exercises, but return to the groove before finishing the pattern.

When exercising the patient's foot, move your proximal hand to a position on the tibia and give resistance to the hip and knee with that hand. Your distal hand is now free to give appropriate resistance to the foot and ankle motions. To avoid fatigue of the hip allow the heel to rest on the table.

> → **Points to remember**
> - **End the pattern with maximal flexion in the knee joint**
> - **Resist the knee flexion with your distal hand throughout the range of motion**
> - **The foot should not move lateral to the knee**

8.2.2 Flexion–Abduction–Internal Rotation
with Knee Extension (Fig. 8.4)

Joint	Movement	Muscles: principal components (Kendall and McCreary 1983)
Hip	Flexion, abduction, internal rotation	Tensor fascia lata, rectus femoris, gluteus medius (anterior), gluteus minimus
Knee	Extension	Quadriceps
Ankle/foot	Dorsiflexion, eversion	Peroneus tertius
Toes	Extension, lateral deviation	Extensor hallucis, extensor digitorum

Position at Start

For this combination place the patient toward the end of the table so the knee can be flexed as fully as possible.

Grip

Your distal and proximal grips remain the same as they were for the straight leg pattern.

Elongated Position

Traction the entire limb as before, while you move the foot into plantar flexion and inversion. Continue the traction while you flex the knee over the end of the table and position the hip in extension with adduction and external rotation. Tightness in the anterior muscles that cross the hip and knee joints may restrict full hip extension–adduction. Keep the thigh in the diagonal and flex the knee only as much as is possible without pain.

 Caution: Do not allow the pelvis to move to the right or go into anterior tilt.

To protect the patient's back, flex the right hip and rest the foot on the end of the table or another support.

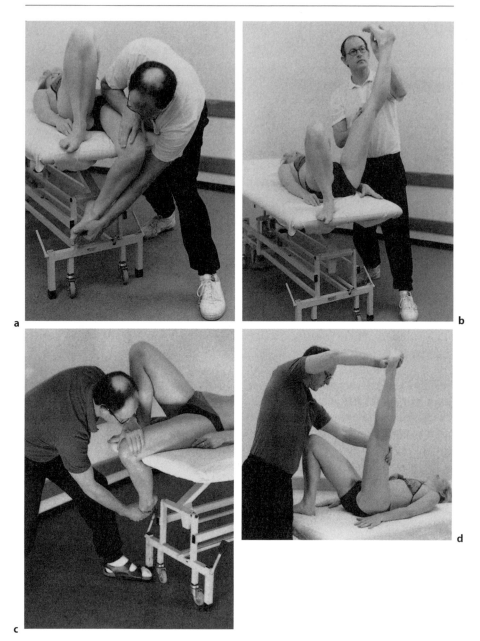

Fig. 8.4a–d. Flexion–abduction–internal rotation with knee extension. **a,b** Usual position of the therapist; **c,d** alternative position at the end of the table

Body Mechanics

Stand in a stride position by the patient's knee. Bend from the hips as you reach down and flex the patient's knee. As the patient lifts his leg with the knee extending your weight shifts back and then you step back.

Alternative Positions

Stand at the end of the table facing up toward the patient's left shoulder. Lean back so that your body weight helps with the stretch of the hip. As the leg moves into flexion, step forward with your back foot (Fig. 8.4 c, d).

Stretch

Apply the stretch to the foot, hip, and knee simultaneously. Stretch the hip with the proximal hand, using rapid traction and rotation. Stretch the foot and ankle with your distal hand, using elongation and rotation. Stretch the knee very gently by applying only traction with your distal hand along the line of the tibia.

Command

"Foot up, bend your hip up and straighten your knee as you go."

Movement

The foot and ankle dorsiflex and evert. The hip motion begins next. When the hip has moved through about $5°$ of flexion the knee begins to extend. It is important that the hip and knee reach their end ranges at the same time.

Resistance

Your distal hand resists the foot and ankle motion with a rotary push. Using the stable foot as a handle, resist the knee extension with a traction force toward the starting position of knee flexion. The rotary resistance at the foot resists the knee and hip rotation as well.

Your proximal hand combines traction through the line of the femur with a twist to resist internal rotation.

! Note: The knee takes more resistance than the hip. Your two hands must work separately.

End Position

The end position is the same as the straight leg pattern.

Timing for Emphasis

The emphasis here is to teach the patient to combine hip flexion with knee extension in a smooth motion.

> → **Points to remember**
> - **Good elongation and rotation in the hip are necessary to facilitate the hip motion**
> - **Do not cause pain with the stretch of the knee**
> - **The hip and knee motions occur together, the end position is a straight leg**

8.3 **Extension–Adduction–External Rotation** (Fig. 8.5)

Joint	Movement	Muscles: principal components (Kendall and McCreary 1983)
Hip	Extension, adduction, external rotation	Adductor magnus, gluteus maximus, hamstrings, lateral rotators
Knee	Extended (positions unchanged)	Quadriceps
Ankle	Plantar-flexion, inversion	Gastrocnemius, soleus, tibialis posterior
Toes	Flexion, medial deviation	Flexor hallucis, flexor digitorum

Grip

Hold the plantar surface of the foot with the palm of your left hand. Your thumb is at the base of the toes to facilitate toe flexion. Be careful not to block the flexion of the toes. Your fingers hold the medial border of the foot, the heel of your hand gives counter-pressure along the lateral border.

> **!** Caution: Do not squeeze or pinch the foot.

Proximal Hand

Your right hand comes underneath the thigh from lateral to medial to hold on the posteromedial side.

Elongated Position

Traction the entire leg while moving the foot into dorsiflexion and eversion. Continue the traction and maintain the internal rotation as you lift the leg into flexion and abduction. If the patient has just completed the antagonistic motion (flexion–abduction–internal rotation), begin at the end of that pattern.

> **!** Caution: Do not try to push the hip past the limitation imposed by hamstring length. Do not allow the pelvis to move into a posterior tilt.

Body Mechanics

Stand in a stride position by the patient's left shoulder facing toward the lower right corner of the table. Your inner foot (closest to the table) is in front. Your weight is on the back foot. Allow the patient's motion to pull you forward onto your front foot. When your weight has shifted over the front foot, step forward with your rear foot and continue the weight shift forward.

Alternative Position

You may stand on the right side of the table facing up toward the left hip. Your right hand is on the plantar surface of the patient's foot, your left hand on the posterior thigh. Stand in a stride and allow the patient to push your weight back as the leg kicks down (Fig. 8.5 d, e).

Stretch

Your proximal hand stretches the hip by giving a quick traction to the thigh. Use the forearm of your distal hand to traction up through the shin while you stretch the patient's foot farther into dorsiflexion and eversion.

 Caution: Do not force the hip into more flexion.

Command

"Point your toes, push your foot down and kick down and in." "Push!"

Movement

The toes flex and the foot and ankle plantar flex and invert. The inversion promotes the hip external rotation, and these motions occur at the same time. The fifth metatarsal leads as the thigh moves down into extension and adduction maintaining the external rotation. Continuation of this motion causes extension with elongation of the left side of the trunk.

Resistance

Your distal hand combines resistance to inversion with approximation through the bottom of the foot. The approximation resists both the plantar flexion and the hip extension. Resisting inversion results in resistance to the hip adduction and external rotation as well. Your proximal hand lifts the thigh back toward the starting position. The lift resists the hip extension and adduction. The placement of your hand, coming from lateral to medial, gives resistance to the external rotation.

As the hip approaches full extension, continue to give approximation through the foot with your distal hand and approximate through the thigh with your proximal hand.

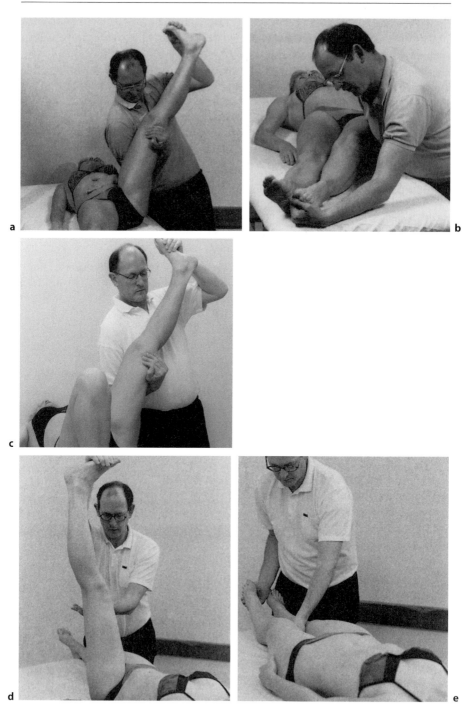

Fig. 8.5 a–e. Extension–adduction–external rotation. **a,b** Therapist standing on the same side of the table; **c** same pattern with the patient's other leg flexed; **d,e** therapist standing on the opposite side of the table

End Position

The foot is in plantar flexion with inversion and the toes are flexed. The knee remains in full extension. The hip is in extension (touching the table) and adduction while maintaining external rotation. The thigh has crossed to the right side of the midline.

Timing for Emphasis

Lock in the hip at the end of the range and exercise the foot and toes.

> → **Points to remember**
> - The therapist's proximal hand comes from the lateral side of the thigh to the posterior-medial surface
> - Normal timing: to get the proper direct movement into the pattern, instead of an arcing movement, the foot must move into its position first
> - End position: the thigh crosses mid-line and the lumbar spine remains in neutral tilt and side bend
> - The hip maintains external rotation as well as adduction

8.3.1 Extension–Adduction–External Rotation with Knee Extension (Fig. 8.6)

Joint	Movement	Muscles: principal components (Kendall and McCreary 1983)
Hip	Extension, adduction, external rotation	Adductor magnus, gluteus maximus, hamstrings, lateral rotators
Knee	Extension	Quadriceps
Ankle	Plantar-flexion, inversion	Gastrocnemius, soleus, tibialis posterior
Toes	Flexion, medial deviation	Flexor hallucis, flexor digitorum

Grip

Your distal and proximal grips are the same as the ones used for the straight leg pattern.

Elongated Position

The foot is in dorsiflexion with eversion. The hip and knee are in full flexion with the heel close to the lateral border of the buttock. The knee and heel are aligned with each other and lined up approximately with the lateral border of the left shoulder. The hip has the same amount of rotation as it did in the straight leg pattern. Straighten the knee to check the rotation.

Body Mechanics

Your body mechanics are the same as for the straight leg pattern.

Alternative Position

You may stand on the opposite side of the table facing up toward the left hip (Fig. 8.6 c, d).

Stretch

Apply the stretch to the hip, knee, and foot simultaneously. With your proximal (right) hand combine traction of the hip through the line of the femur with a rotary motion to stretch the external rotation. Your distal (left) hand stretches the foot farther into dorsiflexion and eversion and stretches the knee extension by bringing the patient's heel closer to his buttock.

> **!** Caution: Don't over-rotate the hip by pulling the foot more lateral than the knee.

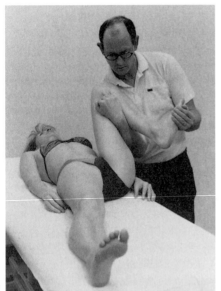
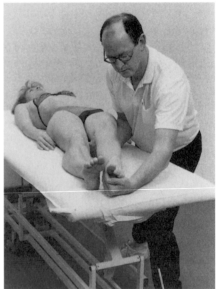
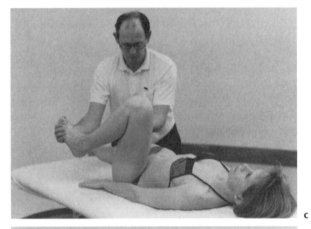
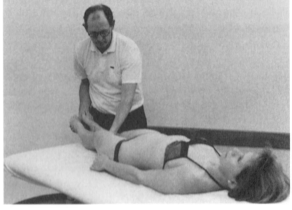

Fig. 8.6 a–d. Extension–adduction–external rotation with knee extension. a, b Usual position of the therapist; c, d alternative position on the other side of the table

Command

"Push your foot down and kick down and in." "Kick!"

Movement

The foot and ankle plantar flex and invert. The hip motion begins next. When the hip extension has completed about $5°$ of motion the knee begins to extend. It is important that the hip and knee reach their end ranges at the same time.

Resistance

Your distal hand resists the foot and ankle motion with a rotary push. The rotary resistance at the foot also resists the rotation at the knee and hip. Using the foot as a handle, resist the knee extension by pushing the patient's heel back toward the buttock. The angle of this resistance will change as the knee moves further into extension. The resistance to the knee extension motion continues in the same direction (toward the patient's buttock) when the knee is fully extended.

Your proximal hand pulls the thigh back toward the starting position. The pull resists the hip extension and adduction. The placement of your hand, coming from lateral to medial, supplies the resistance to the external rotation. As the hip and knee approach full extension, give approximation through the foot with your distal hand and approximate through the thigh with your proximal hand.

Note: The knee takes more resistance than the hip. Your two hands must work separately.

End Position

The end position is the same as the straight leg pattern.

Timing for Emphasis

Prevent knee extension at the beginning of the range and exercise the hip motions. Lock in hip extension in mid-range and exercise the knee extension. Lock in the knee before it is fully extended and exercise the hip extension.

> → **Points to remember**
> - **Don't over-rotate the hip at the beginning of the movement**
> - **Resist the knee extension with your distal hand throughout the range**
> - **Resistance with your distal hand to the knee extension at the beginning of the motion will prevent over rotation of the hip**
> - **The movement ends with external rotation in the hip, not just inversion of the foot**

8.3.2 Extension–Adduction–External Rotation with Knee Flexion (Fig. 8.7)

Joint	Movement	Muscles: principal components (Kendall and McCreary 1983)
Hip	Extension, adduction, external rotation	Adductor magnus, gluteus maximus, lateral rotators
Knee	Flexion	Hamstrings, gracilis
Ankle	Plantar-flexion, inversion	Gastrocnemius, soleus, tibialis posterior
Toes	Flexion, medial deviation	Flexor hallucis, flexor digitorum

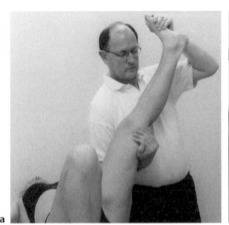 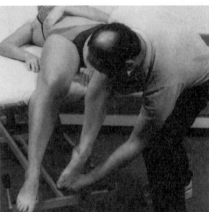

a   b

Fig. 8.7 a, b. Extension–adduction–external rotation with knee flexion

Position at Start

For this combination place the patient toward the end of the table so that the knee can flex as fully as possible. This is the same placement you used to begin the pattern of flexion–abduction–internal rotation with knee extension (Sect. 8.2.2). To protect the patient's back flex the right hip and rest the foot on the end of the table or another support.

Grip

Your distal and proximal grips are the same as those used for the straight leg pattern.

Elongated Position

Position the limb as you did for the straight leg pattern.

Body Mechanics

Use the same body mechanics as for the straight leg pattern. As the pattern nears end range, bend at your hips as you reach down to continue resisting the knee flexion.

Stretch

The stretch comes from the rapid elongation and rotation of the hip, ankle, and foot by both hands simultaneously. With your distal hand you can give increased traction to stretch the knee flexor muscles.

Command

"Push your foot and toes down; push your hip down and bend your knee as you go."

Movement

The foot and ankle plantar flex and invert. The hip motion begins next. When the hip extension has completed about 5° of motion the knee begins to flex. It is important that the hip and knee reach their end ranges at the same time.

Resistance

Your distal hand uses the resistance to the plantar flexion and inversion to resist the knee flexion as well. The pull is back toward the starting position of knee extension and foot eversion. Your proximal hand resists the hip motion as it did for the straight leg pattern. As the hip approaches full extension approximate through the thigh with your proximal hand.

End Position

The hip is extended with adduction and external rotation. The knee is flexed over the end of the table and the foot is in plantar flexion with inversion.

> **!** Caution: Do not allow the pelvis to move to the right or go into anterior tilt.

Timing for Emphasis

Lock in the hip extension at any point in the range and exercise the knee flexion. Do not let the hip action change from extension to flexion. Teach the patient to combine hip extension with knee flexion in a smooth motion.

> → **Points to remember**
> - Resist the flexion of the knee as well as the extension of the hip
> - Normal timing: the knee flexes smoothly during the entire motion
> - Give traction to the femur during the motion

8.4 Flexion–Adduction–External Rotation (Fig. 8.8)

Joint	Movement	Muscles: principal components (Kendall and McCreary 1983)
Hip	Flexion, adduction, External rotation	Psoas major, iliacus, adductor muscles, sartorius, pectineus, rectus femoris
Knee	Extended (position unchanged)	Quadriceps
Ankle/foot	Dorsiflexion, inversion	Tibialis anterior
Toes	Extension, medial deviation	Extensor hallucis, extensor digitorum

Grip

Distal Hand

Your left hand grips the patient's foot with the fingers on the medial border and the thumb giving counter-pressure on the lateral border. Hold the sides of the foot but do not put any contact on the plantar surface. To avoid blocking toe motion, keep your grip proximal to the metatarsal-phalangeal joints. Do not squeeze or pinch the foot.

Proximal Hand

Place your right hand on the anterior-medial surface of the thigh just proximal to the knee.

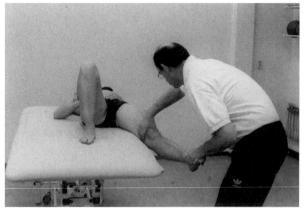

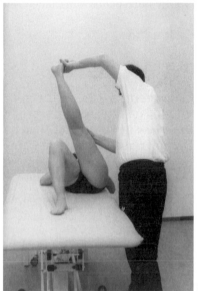

Fig. 8.8a,b. Flexion–adduction–external
rotation

Elongated Position

Traction the entire limb while you move the foot into plantar flexion and
eversion. Continue the traction and maintain the internal rotation as you
place the hip into hyperextension and abduction. The trunk elongates
diagonally from right to left.

> **!** Caution: If the hip extension is restricted, the pelvis will move
> into anterior tilt. If the abduction is restricted, the pelvis will
> move to the left.

Body Mechanics

Stand in a stride position with your inner foot (closest to the table) behind and your outer foot (farthest from the table) in front. Face toward the patient's right shoulder with your body aligned with the pattern's line of motion. Shift your weight from your front foot to your back foot as you stretch. As the patient moves, let the resistance shift your weight forward over your front foot. If the patient's leg is long, you may have to take a step as your weight shifts farther forward. Continue facing the line of motion.

Stretch

The reflex comes from a rapid elongation and rotation of the hip, ankle, and foot by both hands simultaneously.

Command

"Foot up, lift your leg up and in." "Lift up!"

Movement

The toes extend as the foot and ankle move into dorsiflexion and inversion. The inversion promotes the hip external rotation, so these motions occur simultaneously. The big toe leads as the hip moves into flexion with adduction and external rotation. Continuation of this motion produces trunk flexion to the right.

Resistance

Your distal hand combines resistance to inversion with traction through the dorsiflexed foot. The resistance to the hip adduction and external rotation comes from resisting the inversion. The traction resists both the dorsiflexion and hip flexion. Your proximal hand combines traction through the line of the femur with a rotary force to resist the external rotation and adduction. Maintaining the traction force will guide your resistance in the proper arc.

> **!** Caution: Too much resistance to hip flexion may result in strain on the patient's spine.

End Position

The foot is in dorsiflexion with inversion. The knee is in full extension. The hip is in full flexion with enough adduction and external rotation to place the knee and heel in a diagonal line with the right shoulder.

> **!** Caution: The length of the hamstring muscles or other posterior structures may limit the hip motion. Do not allow the pelvis to move into a posterior tilt.

Timing for Emphasis

You may prevent motion in the beginning range of hip flexion and exercise the foot and toes.

> **→** Points to remember
> - Continuation of the lower extremity elongation will tighten the trunk flexors in the same diagonal direction
> - The therapist's body position remains facing the line of motion

8.4.1 Flexion–Adduction–External Rotation with Knee Flexion
(Fig. 8.9)

Joint	Movement	Muscles: principal components (Kendall and McCreary 1983)
Hip	Flexion, adduction, external rotation	Psoas major, iliacus, adductor muscles, sartorius, pectineus, rectus femoris
Knee	Flexion	Hamstrings, gracilis, gastrocnemius
Ankle/foot	Dorsiflexion, inversion	Tibialis anterior
Toes	Extension, medial deviation	Extensor hallucis, extensor digitorum

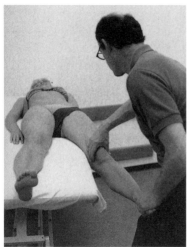
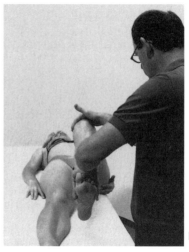
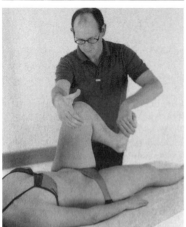

a

b

c

Fig. 8.9 a–c. Flexion–adduction–external rotation with knee flexion

Grip

Your grips are the same as those for the straight leg pattern.

Elongated Position

Position the limb as you did for the straight leg pattern.

Body Mechanics

Stand in the same stride position by the patient's foot as for the straight leg pattern. Again allow the patient to shift your weight from the back to the front foot. Face the line of motion.

Stretch

The reflex comes from a rapid elongation and rotation of the ankle and foot and the hip by both hands simultaneously. Traction with the distal hand facilitates the knee flexors.

Command

"Foot up, bend your leg up and across." "Bend up!"

Movement

The toes extend and the foot and ankle dorsiflex and invert. The hip and knee flexion begin next, and both joints reach their end ranges at the same time. Continuation of this motion also causes trunk flexion to the right.

> Note: Be sure that the knee flexes smoothly and continuously as the hip flexes.

Resistance

Give traction with your proximal hand through the line of the femur, adding a rotary force, to resist the hip motion. The resistance given by your distal hand to the dorsiflexion and inversion will also resist the hip adduction and external rotation. Your distal hand now resists the knee flexion by applying traction through the tibia toward the starting position.

> Note: The resistance to knee flexion is crucial to successful use of this combination for strengthening the hip and trunk.

End Position

The foot is in dorsiflexion with inversion, the hip and knee are in full flexion. The adduction and external rotation cause the heel and knee to line up with each other and with the left shoulder.

Note: An anteroposterior plane bisecting the foot should also bisect the knee. If you extend the patient's knee, the position is the same as the straight leg pattern.

Timing for Emphasis

With three moving segments, hip, knee and foot, you may lock in any two and exercise the third.

With the knee bent it is easy to exercise the external rotation separately from the other hip motions. Do these exercises where the strength of the hip flexion is greatest. You may work through the full range of hip external rotation during these exercises. Return to the groove before finishing the pattern.

When exercising the foot, move your proximal hand to a position on the tibia and give resistance to the hip and knee with that hand. Your distal hand is now free to give appropriate resistance to the foot and ankle motions. To avoid fatigue of the hip allow the heel to rest on the table.

> → **Points to remember**
> - **Normal timing: the knee flexion matches the hip flexion throughout the motion**
> - **There is full flexion of the knee in the end position**
> - **The direction of resistance to the knee flexion is back toward the starting position**
> - **The resistance with the distal hand controls the hip rotation**

8.4.2 Flexion–Adduction–External Rotation with Knee Extension (Fig. 8.10)

Joint	Movement	Muscles: principal components (Kendall and McCreary 1983)
Hip	Flexion, adduction, External rotation	Psoas major, iliacus, adductor muscles, sartorius, pectineus, rectus femoris
Knee	Extension	Quadriceps
Ankle/foot	Dorsiflexion, inversion	Tibialis anterior
Toes	Extension, medial deviation	Extensor hallucis, extensor digitorum

Position at Start

For this combination place the patient closer to the side of the table (Fig. 8.10). An alternative placement is toward the end of the table so that the knee can flex as fully as possible. This is the same placement you used to begin the pattern of flexion–abduction–internal rotation with knee extension (Sect. 8.2.2). To protect the patient's back flex the right hip and rest the foot on the end of the table or another support.

Grip

Your grips remain the same as those for the straight leg pattern.

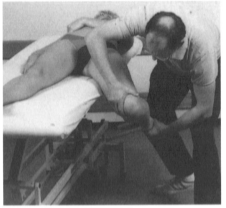
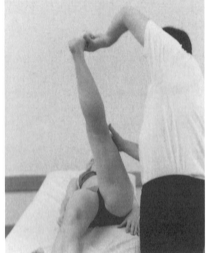

Fig. 8.10 a, b. Flexion–adduction–external rotation with knee extension

Elongated Position

Traction the entire limb as before, while you move the foot into plantar flexion and eversion. Continue the traction on the femur and flex the knee over the side of the table as you position the hip in extension with abduction and internal rotation. Tightness in the anterior muscles that cross the hip and knee joints may restrict full hip extension–abduction. Keep the thigh in the diagonal and flex the knee as much as possible.

 Caution: Do not allow the pelvis to move into anterior tilt. To protect the patient's back flex the right hip and rest the foot on the table or another support.

Body Mechanics

Stand in a stride position by the patient's knee facing the foot of the table. Bend from the hips to reach down and flex the patient's knee. Your weight shifts forward, and then you turn to face the line of the pattern. Step forward as the patient lifts his leg with the knee extending.

Stretch

Apply the stretch to the hip, knee, and foot simultaneously. Stretch the hip with the proximal hand using rapid traction and rotation. Stretch the ankle and foot with your distal hand using elongation and rotation. Stretch the knee very gently by applying only traction with your distal hand along the line of the tibia.

 Caution: Stretch for the knee is traction only. Do not push the knee into more flexion.

Command

"Foot up, bend your hip up and straighten your knee as you go."

Movement

The foot and ankle dorsiflex and invert. The hip motion begins next. When the hip has moved through about 5° of flexion the knee begins to extend. It is important that the hip and knee reach their end ranges at the same time.

Resistance

Your distal hand resists the foot and ankle motion with a rotary force. Using the stable foot as a handle, resist the knee extension with a traction force toward the starting position of knee flexion. The rotary resistance at the foot resists the knee and hip rotation as well.

Your proximal hand combines traction through the line of the femur with a twist to resist the external rotation and adduction.

Note: The knee takes more resistance than the hip. Your two hands must work separately.

End Position

The end position is the same as the straight leg pattern.

Timing for Emphasis

The emphasis here is to teach the patient to combine hip flexion with knee extension in a smooth motion.

→ **Points to remember**
- Elongation in the hip is necessary to facilitate the hip motion
- Do not cause pain with stretch of the knee
- The hip and knee motions occur together
- The end position is a straight leg with adduction and external rotation

8.5 Extension–Abduction–Internal Rotation (Fig. 8.11)

Joint	Movement	Muscles: principal components (Kendall and McCreary 1983)
Hip	Extension, abduction, internal rotation	Gluteus medius, gluteus maximus (upper), hamstrings
Knee	Extended (positions unchanged)	Quadriceps
Ankle	Plantar-flexion, eversion	Gastrocnemius, soleus, peroneus longus and brevis
Toes	Flexion, lateral deviation	Flexor hallucis, flexor digitorum

Grip

Distal Hand

Hold the foot with the palm of your left hand along the plantar surface. Your thumb is at the base of the toes to facilitate toe flexion. Your fingers hold the medial border of the foot while the heel of your hand gives counter pressure along the lateral border.

> **!** Caution: Do not squeeze or pinch the foot.

Proximal Hand

Your right hand holds the posterior lateral side of the thigh.

Elongated Position

Traction the entire leg while moving the foot into dorsiflexion and inversion. Continue the traction and maintain the external rotation as you lift the leg into flexion and adduction.

> **!** Caution: Do not try to push the hip past the limitation imposed by hamstring length. Do not allow the pelvis to move into a posterior tilt.

If the patient has just completed the antagonistic motion (flexion–adduction–external rotation), begin at the end of that pattern.

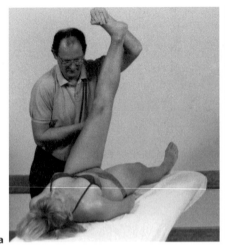
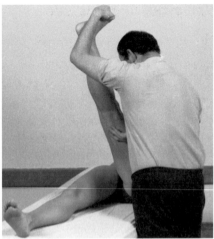

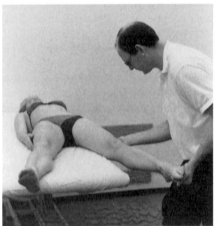

Fig. 8.11 a–c. Extension–abduction–
internal rotation

Body Mechanics

Stand in a stride position facing the patient's right shoulder. Your weight is on
the front foot. Allow the patient to push you back onto your rear foot, then step
back and continue to shift your weight backward. Keep your elbows close to
your sides so you can give the resistance with your body and legs.

Stretch

The proximal hand gives a stretch by rapid traction of the thigh. Use the
forearm of your distal hand to traction up through the shin while you stretch
the patient's foot farther into dorsiflexion and inversion.

> **!** Caution: Do not force the hip into more flexion.

Command

"Point your toes, push your foot down and kick down and out." "Push!"

Movement

The toes flex and the foot and ankle plantar flex and evert. The eversion promotes the hip internal rotation; these motions occur at the same time. The thigh moves down into extension and abduction, maintaining the internal rotation. Continuation of this motion causes extension with left side bending of the trunk.

Resistance

Your distal hand combines resistance to eversion with approximation through the bottom of the foot. The approximation resists both the plantar flexion and the hip extension. The resistance to the hip abduction and internal rotation comes from the resisted eversion. Your proximal hand lifts the thigh back toward the starting position. The lift resists the hip extension and abduction. The placement of your hand, coming from lateral to posterior, gives resistance to the internal rotation.

As the hip approaches full extension, continue to give approximation through the foot with your distal hand and approximate through the thigh with your proximal hand.

End Position

The foot is in plantar flexion with inversion and the toes are flexed. The knee remains in full extension. The hip is in as much hyperextension as possible while maintaining the abduction and internal rotation.

Timing for Emphasis

Use approximation with Repeated Contractions or Combination of Isotonics to exercise the hyperextension hip motion. Lock in the hip at the end of the range and exercise the foot and toes.

→ **Points to remember**
- **Resist the hip extension all the way through the motion**
- **The lumbar spine remains in neutral tilt and side-bend**

8.5.1 Extension–Abduction–Internal Rotation with Knee Extension (Fig. 8.12)

Joint	Movement	Muscles: principal components (Kendall and McCreary 1983)
Hip	Extension, abduction, internal rotation	Gluteus medius, gluteus maximus (upper), hamstrings
Knee	Extension	Quadriceps
Ankle	Plantar-flexion, eversion	Gastrocnemius, soleus, peroneus longus and brevis
Toes	Flexion, lateral deviation	Flexor hallucis, flexor digitorum

Grip

Your grips are the same as for the straight leg pattern.

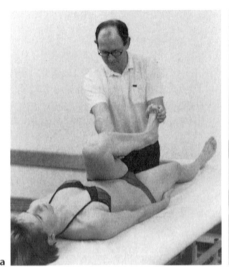
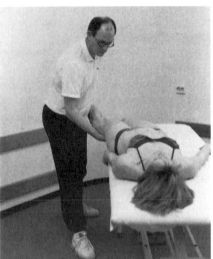

a   b

Fig. 8.12 a, b. Extension–abduction–internal rotation with knee extension

Elongated Position

The foot is in dorsiflexion with inversion. The hip and knee are in full flexion with the heel close to the right buttock. The knee and heel are aligned with each other and lined up approximately with the right shoulder.

Body Mechanics

Your body mechanics are the same as for the straight leg pattern.

Stretch

Apply the stretch to the hip, knee, and foot simultaneously. With your proximal hand combine traction of the hip through the line of the femur with a rotary motion to stretch the internal rotation. Your distal hand stretches the foot farther into dorsiflexion and inversion as you stretch the knee extension by bringing the patient's heel closer to the buttock.

Command

"Push your foot down and kick down and out." "Kick!"

Movement

The foot and ankle plantar flex and evert. The hip motion begins next. When the hip extension has completed about $5°$ of motion the knee begins to extend. It is important that the hip and knee reach their end ranges at the same time.

Resistance

Your distal hand resists the foot and ankle motion with a rotary push. Using the foot as a handle, resist the knee extension by pushing the patient's heel back toward the buttock. The angle of this resistance will change as the knee moves further into extension. The rotary resistance at the foot resists the knee and hip rotation as well.

! Note: The resistance to the knee extension motion continues in the same
• direction when the knee is full extended.

Your proximal hand lifts the thigh back toward the starting position. The lift resists the hip extension and abduction. The placement of the hand from lateral to posterior gives resistance to the internal rotation. As the hip and knee approaches full extension, give approximation through the foot with your distal hand and approximate through the thigh with your proximal hand.

! Note: The knee takes more resistance than the hip. Your two hands must
• work separately.

End Position

The end position is the same as the straight leg pattern.

Timing for Emphasis

Prevent knee extension at the beginning of the range and exercise the hip motions. Lock in hip extension in mid-range and exercise knee extension. Lock in the knee before it is fully extended and exercise the hip extension.

→ **Points to remember**
- **Timing: The hip extends at the same rate as the knee**
- **Your distal hand resists the extension of the knee by pushing the heel toward the buttock**
- **Resistance with your distal hand to the knee extension at the beginning of the motion will prevent over rotation of the hip**

8.5.2 Extension–Abduction–Internal Rotation with Knee Flexion (Fig. 8.13)

Joint	Movement	Muscles: principal components (Kendall and McCreary 1983)
Hip	Extension, abduction, internal rotation	Gluteus medius, gluteus maximus (upper)
Knee	Flexion	Hamstrings, gracilis
Ankle	Plantar-flexion, eversion	Soleus, peroneus longus and brevis
Toes	Flexion, lateral deviation	Flexor hallucis, flexor digitorum

Position at Start

For this combination place the patient closer to the side of the table. This is the same position you used to begin the pattern of flexion–adduction–external rotation with knee extension. To protect the patient's back flex the right hip and rest the foot on the table.

Grip

Your grips are the same as those for the straight leg pattern.

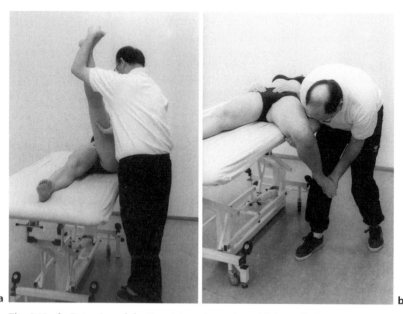

a   b

Fig. 8.13 a, b. Extension–abduction–internal rotation with knee flexion

Elongated Position

Position the limb as you did for the straight leg pattern.

Body Mechanics

Use the same body mechanics as for the straight leg pattern. As the pattern nears end range, bend at your hips as you reach down to continue resisting the knee flexion. You may turn your body to face toward the foot of the table as the knee and hip reach their end range.

Stretch

The reflex comes from the rapid elongation and rotation of the hip, ankle, and foot by both hands simultaneously. You can give a little extra traction movement to the knee with your distal hand to elongate the knee flexor muscles further.

Command

"Push your foot and toes down, push your hip down, and bend your knee as you go."

Movement

The foot and ankle plantar flex and evert. The hip motion begins next. When the hip extension has completed about 5° of motion the knee begins to flex. It is important that the hip and knee reach their end ranges at the same time.

Resistance

Your distal hand resists the plantar flexion and eversion and uses that force to resist the knee flexion as well. The force is back toward the starting position of knee extension and foot inversion. Your proximal hand resists the hip motion as it did for the straight leg pattern. As the hip approaches full extension, approximate through the thigh with your proximal hand.

End Position

The hip is extended with abduction and internal rotation. The knee is flexed over the side of the table and the foot is in plantar flexion with eversion.

 Caution: Do not allow the pelvis to go into anterior tilt.

Timing for Emphasis

Lock in the hip extension at any point in the range and exercise the knee flexion.

 Caution: Do not let the hip action change from extension to flexion.

Teach the patient to combine hip extension with knee flexion in a smooth motion.

→ **Points to remember**
- **Timing: The foot moves first, then the knee and hip move together**
- **End the movement with full hip extension and as much knee flexion as possible without causing lumbar hyperextension**

8.6 Bilateral Leg Patterns

When you exercise both legs at the same time there is always more demand on the trunk muscles than when only one leg is exercising. To exercise the trunk specifically you hold both the legs together. The leg patterns for trunk exercise are discussed in Chapter 10.

When you hold the legs separately the emphasis of the exercise is on the legs. Bilateral leg work allows you to use irradiation from the patient's strong leg to facilitate weak motions or muscles in the involved leg. You can use any combination of patterns and techniques in any position. Work with those patterns, techniques and positions that give you and the patient the greatest advantage in strength and control.

The most common positions for doing bilateral leg patterns are supine, prone, and sitting. In sitting we show two possible combinations. The first is a bilateral symmetrical combination, flexion–abduction with knee extension (Fig. 8.14), and the second is a reciprocal asymmetrical combination, left leg flexion–abduction with knee extension combined with right leg extension–abduction with knee flexion (Fig. 8.15). In a supine position, the symmetrical straight leg combinations of flexion–abduction (Fig. 8.16a,b) and extension–adduction (Fig. 8.16c,d), the reciprocal combination of left leg extension–abduction with right leg flexion–abduction (Fig. 8.17), and the asymmetrical pattern of hyperextension with knee flexion (Fig. 8.18) are shown. In the prone position we show hip extension with knee flexion (Fig. 8.19).

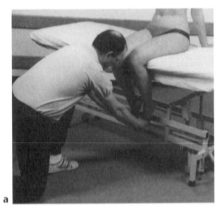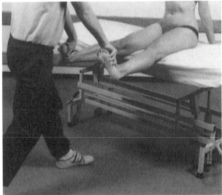

a   b

Fig. 8.14a,b. Bilateral symmetrical pattern combination of flexion–abduction with knee extension in sitting

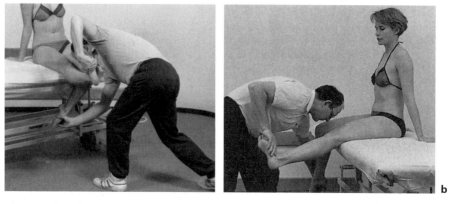

Fig. 8.15 a, b. Bilateral asymmetrical patterns, flexion–abduction with knee extension on the left, extension–abduction with knee flexion on the right

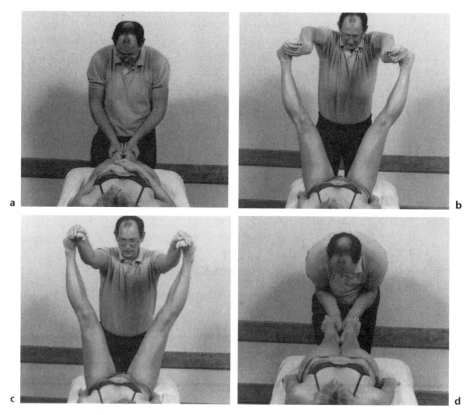

Fig. 8.16 a–d. Bilateral symmetrical combinations in a supine position. **a, b** Flexion-abduction; **c, d** extension–adduction

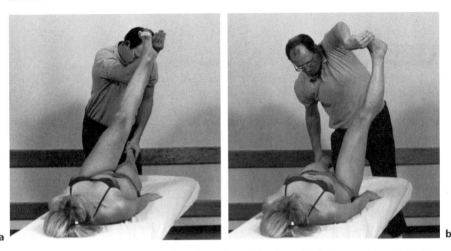

Fig. 8.17 a, b. Bilateral asymmetrical reciprocal combination of left leg extension–abduction with right leg flexion–abduction

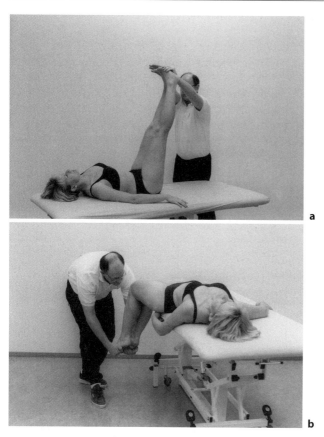

Fig. 8.18 a, b. Bilateral asymmetrical combination of hip extension with knee flexion, left leg in abduction and right leg in adduction

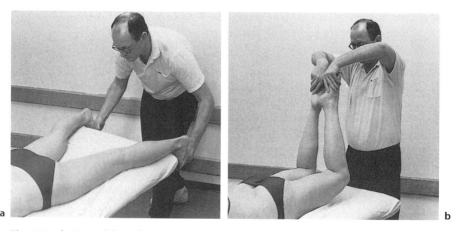

Fig. 8.19 a, b. Prone bilateral symmetrical combination, hip extension–adduction with knee flexion

8.7 Changing the Patient's Position

There are many advantages to exercising the patient in a variety of positions. These include the patient's ability to see his or her leg, adding or eliminating the effect of gravity from a motion, and putting two-joint muscles on stretch. There are also disadvantages for each position. Choose the positions that give the most advantages with the fewest drawbacks. We illustrate four of these positions.

8.7.1 Leg Patterns in a Sitting Position

The sitting position allows the therapist to work with the legs when hip extension is restricted by an outside force. This position lets the patient see the foot and knee while exercising. In addition, working in this position challenges the patient's sitting balance and stability. Using timing for emphasis, this is an easy way to stabilize one leg and exercise the other with reciprocal motions. The number of lower extremity exercises that you can do with your patient in sitting is limited only by the patient's abilities and your imagination. We have pictured three examples in Fig. 8.20.

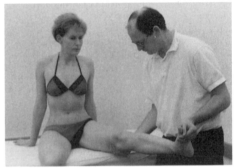

a

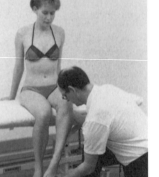

b

Fig. 8.20. Leg patterns in sitting.
a,b Extension–adduction with knee flexion

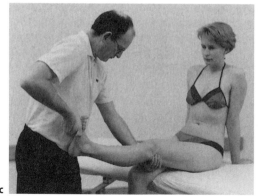

c

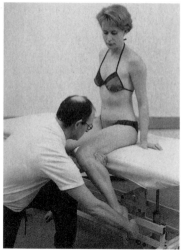

d

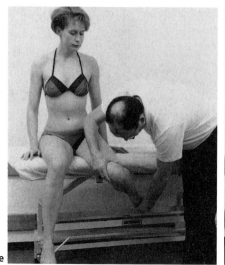

e

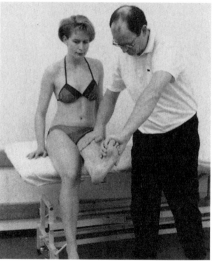

f

Fig. 8.20. Leg patterns in sitting. **c, d** extension–abduction with knee flexion; **e, f** flexion–adduction with knee extension

8.7.2 **Leg Patterns in a Prone Position** (Fig. 8.21a–f)

Working with the patient in a prone position allows you to exercise the hip hyperextension against gravity. This can be good position in which to exercise the combination of hip hyperextension with knee flexion (Fig. 8.21).

Note: Be careful to restrict the motion to the hip. Do not allow the lumbar spine to hyper-extend. To help stabilize the lumbar spine you can position the patient with one leg off the table, hip flexed and foot on the floor (Fig. 8.21 c).

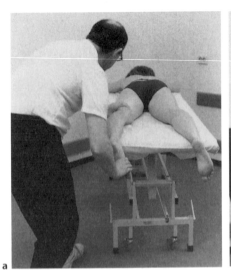
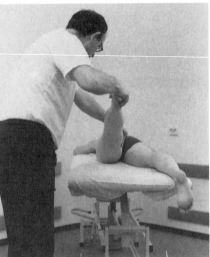

a   b

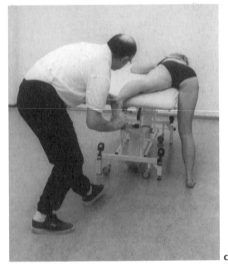

Fig. 8.21. Patterns in prone. a, b Extension–
adduction. c One foot on the floor to
stabilize the lumbar spin

c

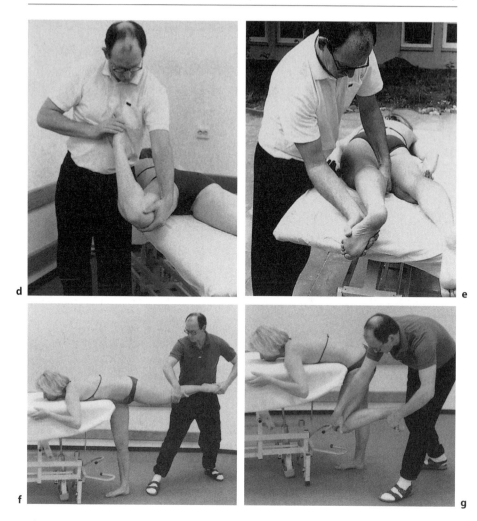

Fig. 8.21. Patterns in prone. **d,e** Flexion-adduction with knee extension. **f,g** Flexion-abduction with knee flexion of the left leg with the right hip flexed and foot on the floor

The table can be used to resist hip flexion when exercising the knee extension with gravity assistance (Fig 8.21d,e).

To exercise hip flexion in a prone position the patient must be positioned with the legs over the end of the table (Fig. 8.21f,g).

8.7.3 Leg Patterns in a Side Lying Position (Fig. 8.22)

When working with the patient in side lying, take care that the patient does not substitute trunk motion or pelvic rolling for the leg motions you want to exercise. You may stabilize the patient's trunk with external support or let the patient do the work of stabilizing the trunk independently. In this position the abductor muscles of the upper leg and the adductor muscles of the lower leg work against gravity. This position is also useful for exercising hip hyperextension. Use approximation and resistance to rotation to facilitate the motion. Resisted posterior depression of the ipsilateral pelvis will help prevent hyperextension of the lumbar spine.

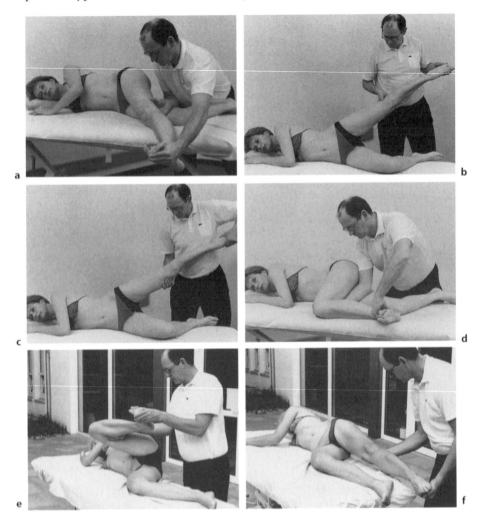

Fig. 8.22. Patterns in side lying. **a,b** Extension–abduction with straight knee; **c,d** flexion–adduction with knee flexion; **e,f** extension–adduction with knee extension

8.7.4 Leg Patterns in a Quadruped Position (Fig. 8.23)

Working in this position requires that the patient stabilizes the trunk and bears weight on the arms as well as on the non-moving leg. As in the prone position, the hip extensor muscles work against gravity. The hip flexion can move through its full range with gravity eliminated.

> **!** Caution: Do not allow the spine to move into undesired positions or postures.

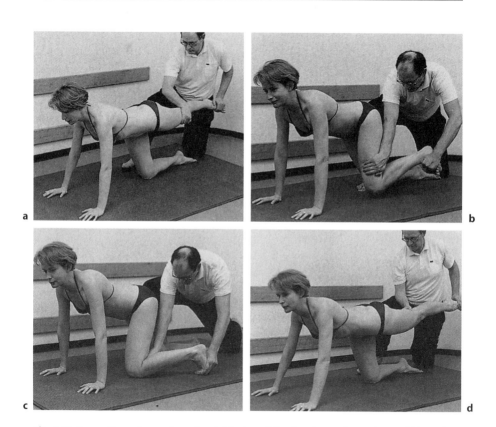

Fig. 8.23. Leg patterns in quadruped. **a, b** Flexion-abduction-internal rotation. **c, d** Extension-adduction-external rotation

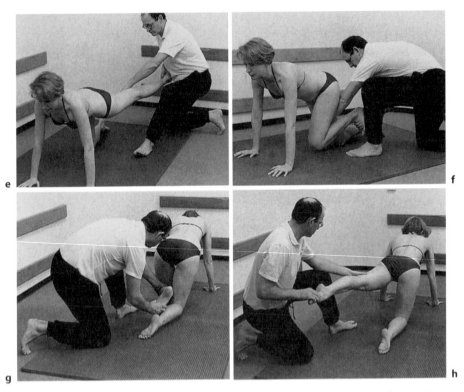

Fig. 8.23. Leg patterns in quadruped. e, f Flexion-adduction-external rotation. g, h Extension-abduction-internal rotation

8.7.5 Leg Patterns in the Standing Position (Fig. 8.24)

Standing or a modified standing position in which patients leans on their hands can be a good position for working with the leg patterns. Resisting the strong leg in flexion–abduction stimulates stability in the hip and knee of the stance leg.

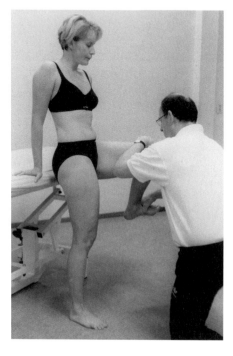

Fig. 8.24. Leg exercise in standing

Reference

Kendall FP, McCreary EK (1983) Muscles, testing and function. Williams and Wilkins, Baltimore

9 The Neck

9.1 Introduction and Basic Procedures

There are many reasons to exercise the neck patterns.

THERAPEUTIC GOALS
- Movement of the head and neck helps to guide trunk motions.
- Resistance to neck motion provides irradiation for trunk muscle exercises.
- You can use the neck patterns when you want to treat dysfunctions in the cervical and thoracic spine directly.
- Stability of the head and neck are essential for most everyday activities.

In this chapter we cover the basic neck patterns and the use of the neck for facilitation of trunk motions.

Diagonal Motion

The neck patterns include the same three motion components as the other patterns: flexion or extension, lateral flexion, and rotation. A plane through the nose, the chin, and the crown of the head defines the proper course of the pattern.

The distal component in the neck patterns is the upper cervical spine. The motion is sometimes called short neck flexion or short neck extension. The proximal component is the lower cervical spine and upper thoracic spine to T6. This motion is sometimes termed long neck flexion or long neck extension.

Movements of the head and eyes reinforce each other. The range of neck motion will be limited if the patient does not look in the direction of the head movement. Giving the patient a specific spot to look at guides the neck motion. Conversely, movement of the head in the appropriate direction facilitates eye motions.

Jaw motion is associated with movement of the head on the neck. Mouth opening and upper cervical flexion reinforce each other. Mouth closing and upper cervical extension reinforce each other.

Irradiation from the neck flexion patterns results in trunk flexion and from the neck extension pattern in trunk elongation. Full neck rotation facilitates trunk lateral flexion.

The neck flexion–extension diagonals are:
- Flexion with right lateral flexion and right rotation, extension with left lateral flexion and left rotation.
- Flexion with left lateral flexion and left rotation, extension with right lateral flexion and right rotation.

In this chapter we illustrate and describe the diagonal of flexion to the left, extension to the right (Fig. 9.1 a, b). To work with the other diagonal, reverse the words "left" and "right" in the instructions. We suggest that you have your patient sitting when you begin practicing the neck patterns.

Table 9.1. Neck Flexion–Lateral Flexion–Rotation

Movement	Muscles: principal components (Kendall and McCreary 1983)
Upper cervical flexion	Longus capitis, rectus capitis anterior, suprahyoid muscles (tuck chin), infrahyoid muscles (stabilize hyoid)
Lower cervical flexion	Longus colli, platysma, scalenus anterior, sternocleidomastoid
Rotation	Contralateral: Scalenus (all), sternocleidomastoid Ipsilateral: Longus capitis and colli, Rectus capitis anterior
Lateral flexion	Longus colli, scalenus (all), sternocleidomastoid

Table 9.2. Neck Extension–Lateral Flexion–Rotation

Movement	Muscles: principal components (Kendall and McCreary 1983)
Upper cervical extension	Iliocostalis and longissimus capitis, obliquus capitis (superior and inferior), rectus capitis posterior (major and minor), semispinalis and splenius capitis, trapezius
Lower cervical extension	Iliocostalis cervicis, longissimus and splenius cervicis, multifidi and rotatores, semispinalis and splenius cervicis, trapezius
Rotation	Contralateral: Multifidi and rotatores, semispinalis capitis, upper trapezius Ipsilateral: Obliquus capitis inferior, splenius cervicis and capitis
Lateral flexion	Iliocostalis cervicis, intertransversarii (cervical), longissimus capitis, obliquus capitis superior, splenius cervicis and capitis, trapezius

Patient Position

Sitting is a functional position for neck motion and stability. In the *prone on elbows* position the neck extensor muscles must work against gravity while neck flexion has gravity assistance. In a *supine position*, neck flexion will assist the patient in rolling and getting to sitting. However, in that position the flexor muscles must be strong enough to lift the head against gravity. *Side lying* eliminates the effects of gravity from the motions of flexion and extension. In this position it is easy to use resisted neck motion to facilitate rolling. Let the purpose of the treatment and the strength of the patient's neck muscles guide you in choosing the correct position. Avoid positions that cause neck pain or general discomfort for the patient.

Therapist Position

To see and control the patient's diagonal neck motion, the best position is on the extension side of center. For example, when the patient moves in the diagonal of right flexion–left extension, stand on the patient's left. For the other diagonal, stand on the patient's right. When the patient is supine or side lying, stand behind the patient. When the patient is prone, sitting, or standing, you may be either in front or behind the patient. Wherever you stand, align your arms and hands with the diagonal motion.

The therapist's body mechanics are essential to guide the head and neck in the right direction. Too little body motion, especially in the extension direction, may lead to decreased cervical extension movement and possibly too much rotation.

Grips

The grips for neck patterns are on the chin and head. The grip on the *chin* controls the upper (short) neck flexion or extension and the rotation. Give the pressure in the center of the chin to avoid side loads on the temporomandibular joint. The grip on the *head* controls the lower (long) neck flexion or extension, the rotation, and the lateral motion. The grip is just a little off center on the side of the lateral motion and rotation with the fingers pointing in the direction of the desired motion.

We find that it is best to grip on the patient's chin with the hand that is on the side of extension. Your other hand goes on the patient's head. The reason for this grip is to keep pressure off the side of the face and the temporomandibular joint.

Example: The patient is sitting and moving in the diagonal of left flexion–right extension. You stand behind the patient on the right (the extension side). Use your right hand on the chin, your left hand on the head.

Example: The patient is prone on elbows and moving in the diagonal of left flexion–right extension. You are standing in front on the patient's right. Use your left hand on the chin, your right hand on the head (Your left hand is on the side of the patient's neck extension because you are facing the patient).

Resistance

Keep the resistance to neck motion within the patient's ability to move or hold without pain or strain. Give resistance to the chin along the line of the mandible. You traction outward to resist flexion and push in to resist extension while resisting the rotation.

Your proximal hand (on the head) resists the rotation, lateral motion and the anterior or posterior motion.

Normal Timing

The normal timing of the neck patterns is from distal (chin motion) to proximal (neck motion). In the flexion and extension patterns, the head moves through the diagonal in a straight line with rotation occurring throughout the motion. The upper cervical spine moves the chin through its full range of flexion (tucking) or extension (lifting) first. The other joints then move the head through the remaining motion. The rotation occurs smoothly throughout the motion.

9.2 Indications

We can use the neck patterns for problems of the trunk (such as hemiplegia, back pain, weakness of the trunk muscles due to various conditions), shoulder problems (such as shoulder-neck syndrome, decreased shoulder range of motion) or for functional problems in walking, rolling, etc.

Neck patterns are used to get irradiation to other parts of our body. For example, for the patient with a total hip replacement resisted neck extension patterns in the supine or prone position will result in irradiation into hip extension and abduction. You can find many ways to use the neck for irradiation to all parts of the body.

You can use the neck patterns to directly treat problems with the cervical spine. However, the PNF philosophy would lead you to start with other stronger and pain free parts of the body such as the pelvis, lower trunk, lower extremities and, when the patient is less acute, the scapula and upper extremities.

> **→ Points to remember**
> - Normal timing is distal (upper cervical) to proximal (lower cervical)
> - Motion in the upper thoracic spine is an essential part of the neck patterns
> - Cervical rotation is an integral part of the patterns. It occurs simultaneously with the other motions

9.3 Flexion to the Left, Extension to the Right (Fig. 9.1)

9.3.1 Flexion/Left Lateral Flexion/Left Rotation (Fig. 9.1 c, d)

Patient Position

The patient is sitting. You are standing behind the patient to the right of center.

Grip

Put the finger tips of your right hand under the patient's chin. Hold the top of the patient's head with your left hand, just left of center. Your left hand and fingers point in the line of the diagonal. Give the resistance with the fingers and palm of that hand. To apply traction with your proximal hand, hook the carpal ridge of your left hand under the patient's occiput and lift in the line of the diagonal.

Elongated Position

The chin is elevated and the neck elongated. The extension is evenly distributed among the cervical and upper thoracic vertebrae. The head is rotated and tilted to the right. The chin, nose, and crown of the head are all on the right side of the patient's midline. You should see and feel that the anterior soft tissues on the left side of the patient's neck are taut. None of the vertebral joints should be in a close-pack position. If you give traction through the neck, the patient's trunk lengthens and rotates to the right.

Body Position and Mechanics

Stand behind the patient, slightly to the right. Your shoulders and pelvis face the diagonal, your arms are aligned with the motion. Allow the patient's motion to pull your weight forward. Allow your body to move slightly forward.

Traction

Apply gentle traction by elongating the entire pattern.

Command

"Tuck your chin in. Bend you head down. Look at your left hip."

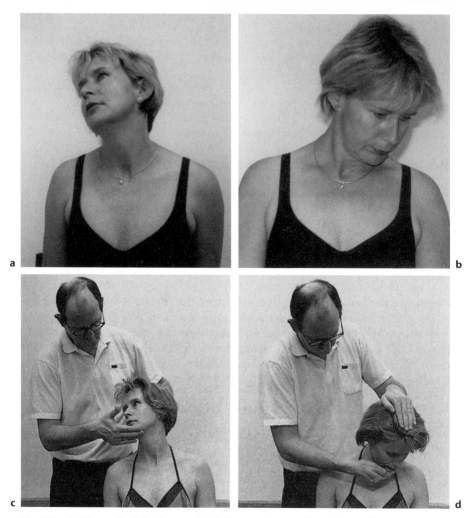

Fig. 9.1 a–d. Diagonal of flexion to the left, extension to the right. **a, b** Active motion through range; **c, d** neck flexion to the left

Movement

The patient's mandible depresses as the chin tucks with rotation toward the left. The neck flexes, following the line of the mandible, bringing the patient's head down towards the chest.

Resistance

Your right hand on the patient's chin gives traction along the line of the mandible and resists the rotation to the left. Your left hand on the patient's head gives a rotational force to the head back toward the starting position.

To give traction with this hand, hook the carpal ridge of your hand under the patient's occiput.

End Position

The patient's head, neck, and upper thoracic spine are fully flexed. The rotation and lateral flexion bring the nose, the chin, and the crown of the head to the left of the midline. The patient's nose points towards the left hip.

Alternative Patient Position

The patient may be prone on the elbows (with the therapist standing behind, Fig. 9.2; or with the therapist standing in front, Fig. 9.3), supine (Fig. 9.4), or in a side lying position (Fig. 9.5).

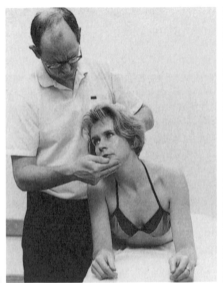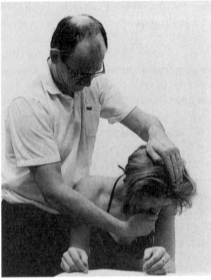

a   b

Fig. 9.2 a, b. Neck flexion to the left, prone on elbows

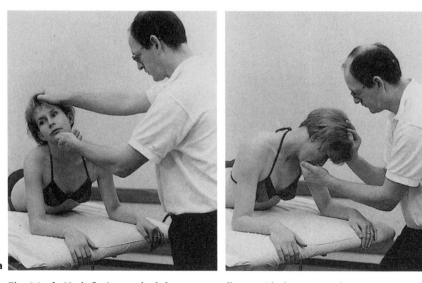

Fig. 9.3 a, b. Neck flexion to the left, prone on elbows with therapist in front

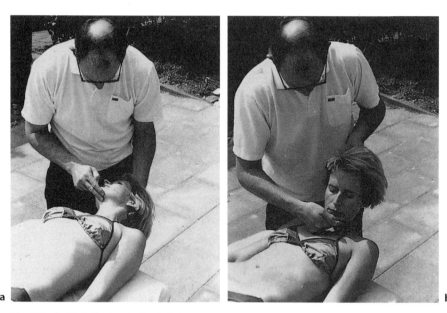

Fig. 9.4 a, b. Neck flexion to the left, in supine

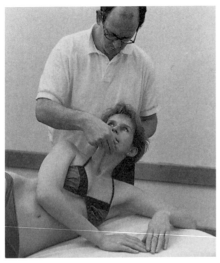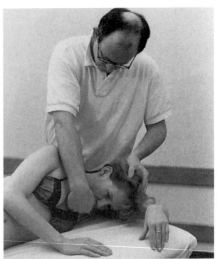

a   b

Fig. 9.5 a, b. Neck flexion to the left, lying on the left side

9.3.2 Extension/Right Lateral Flexion/Right Rotation (Fig. 9.6)

Patient Position

The patient is sitting. You are standing behind the patient to the right of center.

Grip

Put your right thumb on the center of the patient's chin. Hold the top of the patient's head with your left hand, just right of center. Your left hand and fingers point in the line of the diagonal. With this hold, give the resistance with the palm and carpal ridge of your hand. To traction with your proximal hand, hook the carpal ridge under the occiput.

Elongated Position

The chin is tucked and the neck flexed. The head is rotated and tilted to the left. The patient's chin, nose, and crown of the head are all on the left side of the midline. You should see and feel that the posterior soft tissues on the right side of the patient's neck are taut. None of the vertebral joints should be in a close-pack position. If you give traction through the neck, the patient's trunk flexes and rotates to the left.

Body Position and Mechanics

Stand behind the patient, slightly to the right. Your shoulders and pelvis face the diagonal, your arms are aligned with the motion. Allow the patient's motion to push your weight back, and allow your body to move away from the patient.

Traction

Apply gentle traction to the skull to elongate the neck. Gently compress on the chin through the line of the mandible.

Command

"Lift your chin. Lift your head. Look up."

Movement

The patient's mandible protrudes and the chin lifts with rotation toward the right. The neck and upper thoracic spine extend, following the line of the mandible. The patient's neck and upper spine elongate as the head comes up.

Resistance

Your right hand on the patient's chin compresses along the line of the mandible and resists rotation to the right. Your left hand on the patient's head gives a rotational force to the head back toward the starting position. Use traction through the head during the first part of the motion. As the neck approaches the extended position, you may apply gentle compression through the top of the patient's head.

End Position

The patient's head, neck, and upper thoracic spine are extended with elongation. The rotation and lateral flexion bring the nose, the chin, and the crown of the head to the right of the midline.

> **!** Caution: Do not allow excessive extension in the mid-cervical area. The neck must elongate, not shorten.

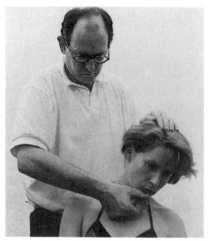 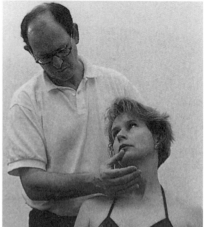

a   b

Fig. 9.6a,b. Neck extension to the right in sitting

Alternative Patient Positions

The patient may be prone on the elbows with the therapist standing behind (Fig. 9.7) or standing in front, supine, or in a side lying position.

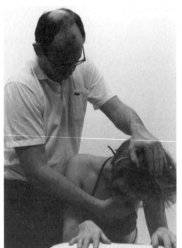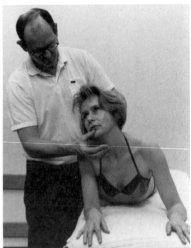

a   b

Fig. 9.7 Neck extension to the right, prone on elbows

9.4 Neck for Trunk

When the neck is strong and pain-free you can use it as a handle to exercise the trunk muscles. Both static and dynamic techniques work well. If there is a chance that motion will cause pain, pre-position the neck in the desired end range and use static contractions.

Note: The head and neck are the handle, the action happens in the trunk.

When using neck flexion patterns, the main component of resistance is traction. With extension patterns, gentle compression through the crown of the head will facilitate trunk elongation with the extension.

9.4.1 Neck for Trunk Flexion and Extension

With the patient supine, use the neck to facilitate rolling forward (Fig. 9.8 a, b). If the patient has good potential trunk strength use the neck to facilitate a supine-to-sitting motion. With the patient side lying or prone use neck extension to facilitate rolling back (Fig. 9.8 c). Resist static neck flexion and extension patterns with the patient's head in the midline to facilitate static contractions of the trunk muscles in sitting. To challenge the patient's sitting balance use reversal techniques, either static or with small reversing motions.

When you exercise the patient in standing give gentle resistance to the neck patterns. Combine this with resistance at the shoulder or pelvis.

→ **Points to remember**
- **The head and neck are the handle to facilitate trunk activity**
- **You can use one hand to resist the scapula or pelvis**

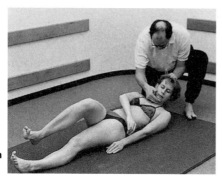
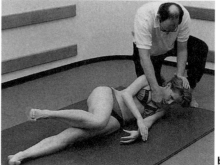

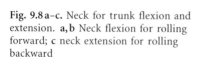

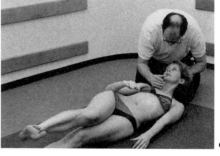

Fig. 9.8 a–c. Neck for trunk flexion and extension. **a, b** Neck flexion for rolling forward; **c** neck extension for rolling backward

9.4.2 Neck for Trunk Lateral Flexion

This activity can be used in all positions. The shortening on the working side results in concurrent lengthening on the other side. The trunk lateral flexion is facilitated by the chin tuck (upper cervical flexion), rotation, and lateral flexion. The head is positioned actively by the patient. After the head is in position all further motion occurs in the trunk. This exercise can be done with a flexion or an extension bias.

> → **Points to remember**
> - **The head and neck are the handle to facilitate the trunk activity**
> - **The head and neck position are pain-free**

The basic combination of neck motions for trunk lateral flexion are:
- Full cervical rotation
- Ipsilateral lateral flexion
- Upper cervical (short neck) flexion
- Lower cervical (long neck) extension

Neck for Right Lateral Trunk Flexion with Flexion Bias
(Fig. 9.9 a–c)

Begin with the patient's chin tucked and the head turned so that the chin aims towards the front of the right shoulder.

Body Position and Mechanics

Stand at the patient's left side, opposite to the direction of rotation.

Grip

Place your right hand on the right side of the patient's head (by the right ear). Put left hand under the patient's chin.

Alternative Body Position and Grip

Stand so the patient turns towards you. Put your left hand by the patient's right ear. Place the fingers of your right hand under the patient's chin.

Command (Preparation)

"Turn your head to the right and put your chin here (touching the front of the right shoulder)."

Command

"Keep your chin on your shoulder, don't let me move your head." "Now pull your chin farther to your shoulder" "Now do it again."

Resistance

Your distal hand (chin) resists upper (short) neck flexion, rotation and lateral flexion. Your proximal hand resists lower (long) neck extension, rotation and lateral flexion.

Motion

The upper trunk side-bends to the right, the right shoulder moves towards the right ilium. The motion includes flexion and right rotation.

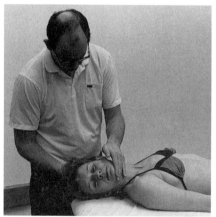

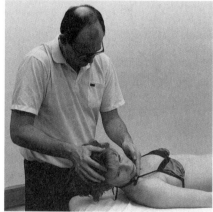

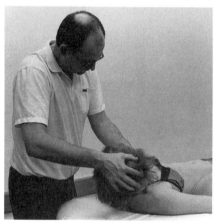

Fig. 9.9. Neck for trunk right lateral flexion. a–c In supine with flexion bias

Neck for Right Lateral Trunk Flexion with Extension Bias
(Fig. 9.9 d, e)

Begin with the patient's chin tucked and the head turned so the chin aims toward the back of the right shoulder.

Body Position and Mechanics

Stand at the patient's left side opposite to the direction of rotation.

Grip

The grip is the same as before.

Alternative Body Position and Grip

These are the same as before.

Command (Preparation)

"Turn your head to the right and try to put your chin behind your right shoulder."

Command

"Keep your chin on your shoulder and your ear back; don't let me move your head." "Now pull your chin farther behind your shoulder." "Now do it again."

Resistance

Your distal hand (chin) resists the upper (short) neck flexion, rotation and lateral flexion. Your proximal hand resists lower (long) neck extension, rotation, and lateral flexion.

Note: When your patient is prone, the rotational resistance is away from you (toward the front of the patient). Therefore, your left hand grips the head, your right hand grips the chin.

Motion

The upper trunk side-bends to the right with extension, the right shoulder moves toward the back of the right ilium. The motion includes trunk extension and right rotation (Fig. 9.9 d–f).

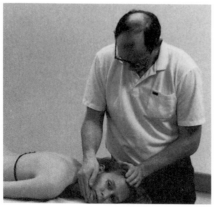

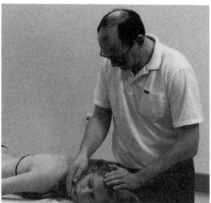

d   e

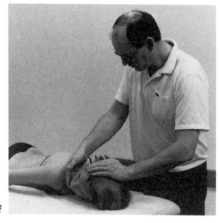

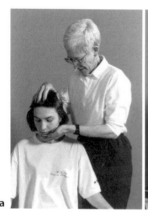

f

Fig. 9.9. Neck for trunk right lateral flexion. **d–f** in prone with extension bias

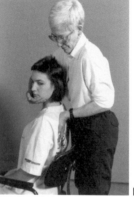

a   b

Fig. 9.10 a, b. Patient with incomplete tetraplegia after a traumatic fracture C2 and C6. **a** Flexion, lateral flexion and rotation to the right. **b** Timing for emphasis with neck rotation to the left for good trunk extension to the left

Reference

Kendall FP, McCreary EK (1983) Muscles, testing and function. Williams and Wilkins, Baltimore

10 The Trunk

10.1 Introduction and Basic Procedures

A strong trunk is essential for good function. The trunk is the base that supports extremity motions. For example, supporting trunk muscles contract synergistically with arm motions (Angel and Eppler 1967). This is often clear in patients with neurologic problems. When the trunk is unstable, normal movement in the extremities is impossible. With the trunk able to move and stabilize effectively, patients gain improved control of their arms and legs.

Strengthening the muscles of the trunk is only one reason for using the trunk patterns in patient treatment. Some other uses for these patterns are:
- Resisting the lower trunk patterns provides irradiation for indirect treatment of the neck and scapular muscles.
- Continuing the upper trunk patterns exercises the patient's hips by moving the pelvis on the femur.
- Resisted trunk activity will produce irradiation into the other extremities. For example, when you resist the lower extremities for trunk flexion and extension, the patient's arm muscles work to help with stabilization.

Use of the scapula and pelvis to facilitate activity of the trunk muscles is covered in Chap. 6. Chapter 9 describes using the neck to facilitate trunk motion. In this chapter we focus on using the extremities to exercise the trunk muscles. The emphasis is on the trunk when the arms are joined by one hand gripping the other arm or when the legs are touching and move together.

Diagonal Motion

The trunk flexion and extension patterns have the same three motion components as the other patterns: flexion or extension, lateral flexion, and rotation. The axis of motion for the flexion and extension patterns runs approximately from the coracoid process to the opposite anterior superior iliac spine (ASIS). The lateral flexion (side-bending) patterns have three components as well. The emphasis in this activity is lateral trunk bending with accompanying rotation and flexion or extension.

We consider the rotation to be of the entire upper or lower trunk, not of the individual spinal segments. Therefore, upper trunk left rotation is the motion of bringing the right shoulder toward the left ilium. Left rotation of the lower trunk brings the right ilium towards the left shoulder.

Table 10.1. Trunk Flexion to the Left–Left Lateral Flexion–Left Rotation of the Trunk

Movement	Muscles: principal components (Kendall and McCreary 1983)
Chopping to the left	Left external oblique, rectus abdominis, right internal oblique
Bilateral lower extremity flexion to the left	Left internal oblique, rectus abdominis, right external oblique

Table 10.2. Trunk Extension to the Right-Right Lateral Flexion–Right Rotation of the Trunk

Movement	Muscles: principal components (Kendall and McCreary 1983)
Lifting to the right	All the neck and back extensor muscles, left multifidi and rotatores
Bilateral lower extremity extension to the right	All the back and neck extensor muscles, Right quadratus lumborum, Left multifidi and rotatores

Table 10.3. Trunk Lateral Flexion to the Right (Right Side Bending)

Movement	Muscles: principal components (Kendall and McCreary 1983)
With extension bias	Quadratus lumborum, iliocostalis lumborum, Longissimus thoracis, latissimus dorsi (when arm is fixed)
With flexion bias	Right internal oblique, right external oblique

In this chapter we illustrate and describe the diagonal of flexion to the left, extension to the right. To work with the other diagonal, reverse the words "left" and "right" in the instructions.

Patient Position

The patient can be in any position when exercising the trunk muscles. We have found that the following combinations give good results:
- Supine: upper and lower trunk flexion and extension, lateral flexion
- Side lying: upper and lower trunk flexion and extension
- Prone: upper trunk extension, lateral flexion
- Sitting: upper trunk flexion and extension, upper trunk side bending using the neck, irradiation from the upper trunk into lower trunk and hip motions

We introduce the patterns with the patient supine and show variations of position later in the chapter.

Resistance

Block the initial motion of the extremities until you feel or see the patient's trunk muscles contract. Then allow the extremities to move, maintaining enough resistance to keep the trunk muscles contracting.

Normal Timing

With these combination patterns, the extremities start the motion while the trunk muscles stabilize. After the extremities have moved through range, the trunk completes its motion.

Timing for Emphasis

Lock in the extremities at the end of their range of motion. Use them as a handle to exercise the trunk motion.

10.2 Chopping and Lifting

These combination patterns use bilateral, asymmetrical, upper extremity patterns combined with neck patterns to exercise trunk muscles. The arms are resisted as a unit. Successful use of these combinations requires that at least one arm must be strong.

Note: You may use any elbow motion with the shoulder patterns. We have used the straight arm patterns in these illustrations.

10.2.1 Chopping

Bilateral asymmetrical upper extremity extension with neck flexion is used for trunk flexion, as shown here. Other uses for the chopping pattern are:
- Facilitating functional motions such as rolling forward or coming to sitting
- Exercising hip flexion when the muscles of trunk flexion are strong

Chopping to the left is illustrated in Fig. 10.1, and Fig. 10.2. Its components are:
- Left arm (the lead arm): extension–abduction–internal rotation
- Right arm (the following arm): extension–adduction–internal rotation. The following (right) hand grips the lead (left) wrist
- Neck: flexion to the left

Patient Position

The patient is supine and close to the left side of the table.

Body Position and Mechanics

Stand in a stride position on the left side of the table facing toward the patient's hands. This is the same position used to resist the single arm pattern of extension–abduction–internal rotation. Let the patient's motion push your weight back. As the patient's arm nears the end of the range, turn your body so you face the patient's feet.

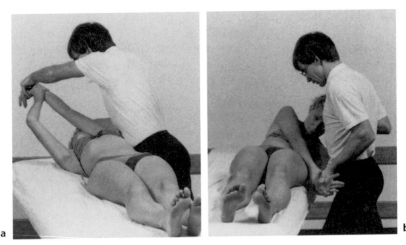

Fig. 10.1 a, b. Chopping to the left in supine

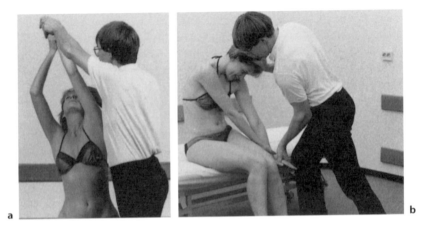

Fig. 10.2 a, b. Chopping to the left in sitting

Grip

Distal Hand

Your left hand grips the patient's left hand (leading hand). Use the normal distal grip for the pattern of extension–abduction–internal rotation.

Proximal Hand

Place your right hand on the patient's forehead with your fingers pointing toward the crown.

Elongated Position

The patient's left arm is in flexion–adduction–external rotation. The right hand grips the left wrist with the right arm in modified flexion–abduction–external rotation. The patient looks at the left hand, putting the neck in modified extension to the right (Fig. 10.1 a).

Stretch

Traction the left arm and scapula until you feel the trunk muscles elongate. Continue the traction to give stretch to the arms and the trunk.

Command

"Push your arms down to me and lift your head. Now keep your arms down here and push some more." "Reach for your left knee."

Movement

The patient's left arm moves through the pattern of extension–abduction–internal rotation with the right arm following into extension–adduction–internal rotation. The patient's head and neck come into flexion to the left. At the same time, the patient's upper trunk begins to move into flexion with rotation and lateral flexion to the left.

Resistance

The major resistance is to the arm motion and through the arms into the trunk. The resistance to the head is light and serves mainly to guide the head and neck motion.

Use resistance to hold back on the beginning arm motion until you feel and see the abdominal muscles begin to contract. Then allow the arms and head to complete their motion against enough resistance to keep the trunk flexor muscles contracting. As the trunk begins to flex, add approximation through the arms.

End Position

The left arm is extended by the patient's side and the patient's neck is in flexion to the left. The upper trunk is flexed to the left as far as the patient can go.

Normal Timing

The abdominal muscles begin to contract as soon as the arms and head begin their motion. By the time the arms and head have finished their movement, the upper trunk is flexed with left rotation and left lateral flexion.

Timing for Emphasis

Lock in the arms at their end range using approximation and rotational resistance. Using the stable arms as a handle, exercise the trunk flexion.

Note: In the end position the arms and head are the handle and do not move. Only the trunk moves as you exercise it.

When working on the mats use chopping to help the patient roll forward or go from supine to sitting. The rotational resistance and approximation through the arms promote and resist the patient's movement to sitting. Shift the angle of resistance slightly to the side to get the patient to roll.

Alternative Position

Sitting

Your goal can be flexion of the trunk with gravity assistance or flexion of the hips with irradiation from the arms and trunk. Use this position to train the trunk and hip flexor muscles in eccentric work.

→ **Points to remember**
- **At the end of the pattern only the trunk moves, the arms are the handle**
- **The proximal hand can resist the contralateral scapular motion of anterior-depression**

10.2.2 Lifting

Bilateral asymmetrical upper extremity flexion with neck extension is used for trunk extension, as shown here. Other uses for the lifting pattern are:
- Exercising hip extension when the trunk extensor muscles are strong
- Facilitating functional motions such as rolling backward or coming to erect sitting from a slumped position.

Lifting to the left is illustrated in Fig. 10.3. Its components are:
- Left arm (the lead arm): flexion–abduction–external rotation
- Right arm (the following arm): flexion–adduction–external rotation. The following (right) hand grips the lead (left) wrist
- Neck: extension to the left

Patient Position

The patient is supine and close to the left side of the table (Fig. 10.3 a, b).

Body Position and Mechanics

Stand in a stride position at the head of the table on the left side facing toward the patient's hands. Let the patient's motion push your weight back. As the patient's arm nears the end of the range, step back in the line of the diagonal.

Grip

Distal hand

Your left hand grips the patient's left hand (leading hand). Use the normal distal grip for the pattern of flexion–abduction–external rotation.

Proximal hand

Place your right hand on the crown of the patient's head with your fingers pointing toward the left side of the patient's neck.

Elongated Position

The patient's left arm is in extension–adduction–internal rotation. The right hand grips the left wrist with the right arm in modified extension–abduction–internal rotation. The patient looks at the left hand putting the neck in flexion to the right (Fig. 10.3 a).

Stretch

Traction the left arm and scapula until you feel the arm and trunk muscles elongate. Continue the traction to give stretch to the arms and the trunk. Traction the patient's head to elongate the neck extensor muscles.

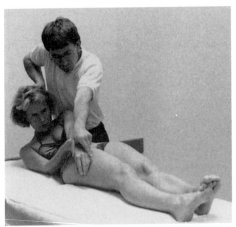
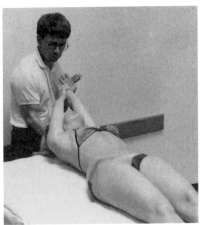
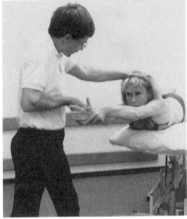
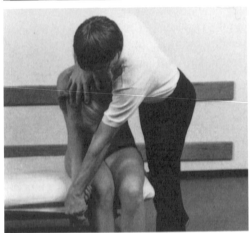
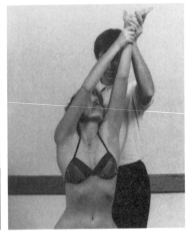

a   b

c

d   e

Fig. 10.3 a–e. Lifting: a,b lifting to the left in supine; c lifting to the right in prone; d,e lifting to the left in sitting

Command

"Lift your arms up to me and push your head back. Follow your hands with your eyes. Now keep your arms and head back here and push some more."

Movement

The patient's left arm moves through the pattern of flexion–abduction–external rotation with the right arm following into flexion–adduction–external rotation. The patient's head and neck come into extension to the left. At the same time the patient's upper trunk begins to move into extension with rotation and lateral flexion to the left.

Resistance

The resistance is to the arm and head motion and through them into the trunk. Use resistance to hold back on the beginning arm and head motion until you feel and see the back extensor muscles begin to contract. Then allow the arms and head to complete their motion against enough resistance to keep the trunk extensor muscles contracting.

End Position

The arms are fully flexed with the left arm by the patient's left ear. The patient's head is extended to the left. The trunk is extended and elongated to the left. The extension continues down to the legs if the patient's strength permits.

Normal Timing

The back extensor muscles begin to contract as soon as the arms and head begin their motion. By the time the arms and head have finished their movement the trunk is elongated to the left with left rotation and slight left lateral flexion.

Timing for Emphasis

Lock in the arms and head at their end range. Lock in the arms using resistance to rotation and approximation, the neck with resistance to rotation and extension. Use the arms and head as a handle to exercise the trunk extension (elongation). Neither the arms nor the head should move while the trunk is exercising. Use lifting when the patient is lying on the mats with the goal of rolling backward.

Alternative Positions

Prone

Exercise in the end range against gravity. This position is particularly good with stronger and heavier patients (Fig. 10.3 c).

Sitting

Your goal is elongation of the trunk. Do not allow the patient to move into hyper lordosis in the cervical or lumbar spine.

Use lifting to facilitate moving from a bent (flexed) to an upright (extended) position. Lifting is also good for teaching the patient erect posture (Fig. 10.3 d, e).

> ➡ **Points to remember**
> - At the end of the pattern only the trunk moves, the arms are the handle
> - The desired activity is trunk elongation, not lumbar spine hyperextension

10.3 Bilateral Leg Patterns for the Trunk

These combinations use bilateral, asymmetrical, lower extremity patterns to exercise trunk muscles. Hold the legs together and resist them as a unit. Successful use of these combinations requires that at least one leg be strong.

Note: You may use any knee motion with the hip patterns. The usual combination is hip flexion with knee flexion and hip extension with knee extension.

10.3.1 Bilateral Lower Extremity Flexion, with Knee Flexion, for Lower Trunk Flexion (Right) (Fig. 10.4)

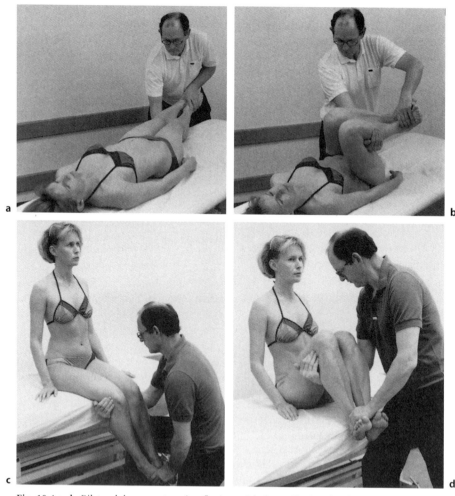

Fig. 10.4a–d. Bilateral lower extremity flexion with knee flexion for lower trunk flexion. a, b Supine; c, d sitting

Position at Start

Position the patient close to the edge of the table. The patient's legs are together with the left leg in extension–abduction–internal rotation and the right leg in extension–adduction–external rotation.

Body Mechanics

Stand in a stride facing the diagonal. Lean back to elongate and stretch the pattern. As the patient's legs move up into flexion, step forward with your rear leg. Use your body weight to resist the motion.

Grip

Distal hand

Your left hand holds both of the patient's feet with contact on the dorsal and lateral surfaces of both feet. Do not put your finger between the patient's feet. If the feet are too large for your grasp, cross one foot partially over the other to decrease the width.

Proximal hand

Your right arm is underneath the patient's thighs. Hold the thighs together with this arm.

Elongated Position

The trunk is extended and elongated to the left with left rotation and side-bending.

> **!** Caution: Avoid hyperextension in the lumbar spine.

Stretch

Traction and rotate the legs to elongate and stretch the lower extremity and trunk flexor muscles.

Note: Do not pull the lumbar spine into hyperextension.

Command

"Feet up, bend your legs up and away. Bring your knees to your right shoulder."

Movement

As the feet dorsiflex the trunk flexor muscles begin to contract. The legs flex together, the right leg into flexion–abduction–internal rotation, the left leg into flexion–adduction–external rotation. When the legs reach the end of their range, the motion continues as lower trunk flexion with rotation and side-bending to the right.

Resistance

Distal Hand

This hand resists the trunk and hip rotation with traction back toward the starting position. Resist the knee motion with this hand as you did with the single leg patterns. If the knees remain straight, give traction through the line of the tibia. If using knee flexion, resistance to that motion will control the trunk.

Proximal Hand

Continue to hold the thighs together with this arm. Use your hand to resist rotation and lateral motion with pressure on the lateral border of the thigh. Give traction through the line of the femur.

> **! Caution:** Too much resistance to hip flexion will cause the lumbar spine to hyperextend.

Library Services
University of Birmingham

Circulation system messages:
Patron in file

Title: Proprioceptive neuromuscular
facilitation :
ID: 5517835968
Due: 25/02/2014 23:59
Circulation system messages:
Loan performed

Title: PNF in practice :
ID: 5523074019
Due: 25/02/2014 23:59
Circulation system messages:
Loan performed

Title: Vestibular rehabilitation /
ID: 5525410458
Due: 25/02/2014 23:59
Circulation system messages:
Loan performed

Total items: 3
28/01/2014 16:16

If you don't like long queues or
paying fines, please renew or return
your short loan items between 8.30-
11.00am.

Library Services
University of Birmingham

Circulation system messages
Patron in file

Title: Proprioceptive neuromuscular facilitation :
ID: SS17838968
Due: 26/02/2014 23:59
Circulation system messages
Loan performed

Title: PNF in practice :
ID: SS23074019
Due: 26/02/2014 23:59
Circulation system messages
Loan performed

Title: Vestibular rehabilitation /
ID: SS25410458
Due: 26/02/2014 23:59
Circulation system messages
Loan performed

Total items: 3
28/01/2014 16:10

If you don't like long queues or paying fines, please renew or return your short loan items before 9.30.
11.03am

End Position

The right leg is in full flexion–abduction–internal rotation, the left leg in full flexion–adduction–external rotation. The lower trunk is flexed with rotation and lateral flexion to the right.

Normal Timing

As soon as or just before the feet begin to dorsi-flex the trunk flexor muscles contract. After the hips have reached their end range, the motion continues with lower trunk flexion.

> **!** Caution: Do not allow the lumbar spine to be pulled into hyper-extension. Start with the legs flexed if the trunk flexor muscles cannot stabilize the pelvis at the beginning of the motion.

Timing for Emphasis

Lock in the lower extremities in their end position. Use the legs as a handle to exercise the trunk motion. You may use static or dynamic exercises.

! Note: In the end position the legs are the handle. Only the pelvis moves while you exercise the trunk. The pivot of emphasis can be changed to trunk lateral flexion. See Sect. 10.3.3.

To exercise neck and upper trunk flexion, use prolonged static contraction of the legs and lower trunk muscles. Using the legs and lower trunk in this way works well when the patient's arms are too weak to use for upper trunk exercise. This combination is also useful when the patient has pain in the neck or upper trunk.

Alternative Positions

Use this lower extremity combination on the mats to facilitate rolling from supine to side-lying or in the short sitting position (Fig. 10.4 c, d).

> **→** Points to remember
> - The lumbar spine must not be pulled into hyperextension
> - The legs become the handle; only the pelvis moves to exercise the trunk

10.3.2 Bilateral Lower Extremity Extension, with Knee Extension, for Lower Trunk Extension (Left) (Fig. 10.5)

Position at Start

Position the patient close to the left side of the table.

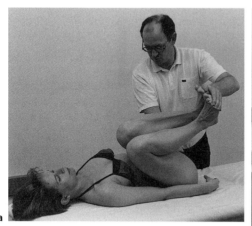
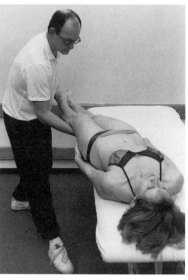

Fig. 10.5 a, b. Bilateral lower extremity extension with knee extension for lower trunk extension

Body Mechanics

Stand in a stride position facing the diagonal. Lean forward to stretch the pattern. As the patient's legs move into extension, step back with your forward leg. Use your body weight to resist the motion.

Grip

Distal Hand

Your left hand holds both of the patient's feet with contact on the plantar and lateral surfaces close to the toes. If the feet are too large for your grasp, cross one foot partially over the other to decrease the width.

Proximal Hand

Your right arm is underneath the patient's thighs. Hold the thighs together with this arm.

Elongated Position

The patient's legs are flexed to the right. The right leg is in flexion–abduction–internal rotation with knee flexion, the left leg in flexion–adduction–external rotation with knee flexion. The lower trunk is flexed with rotation and lateral flexion to the right.

Stretch

Use traction with rotation through the thighs to increase the trunk flexion to the right.

Command

"Toes down, kick down to me."

Movement

As the feet plantar flex the trunk extensor muscles begin to contract. The legs extend together, the left leg into extension–abduction–internal rotation, right leg into extension–adduction–external rotation. When the legs reach the end of their range, the motion continues as lower trunk elongation with rotation and side-bending to the left.

Resistance

Distal Hand

Resist trunk and hip rotation with pressure on the feet. Resist the knee extension with this hand as you did with the single leg patterns by pushing the patient's heels back toward the buttock. Resistance with your distal hand to the knee extension at the beginning of the motion will prevent over rotation of the hips and trunk.

If the knees remain straight, give approximation through the line of the tibia.

Proximal Hand

Continue to hold the thighs together with this arm as you resist the hip motions.

End Position

The left leg is in full extension–abduction–internal rotation, the right leg in full extension–adduction–external rotation. The lower trunk is elongated with rotation and lateral flexion to the left.

Normal Timing

The trunk extensor muscles contract as soon as or just before the legs begin their motion. By the time the leg motion is completed the trunk is in full elongation.

> **!** Caution: The end position is trunk elongation, not lumbar spine hyperextension.

Timing for Emphasis

To exercise the neck and upper trunk extension, use prolonged static contraction of the legs and lower trunk muscles. Using the legs and lower trunk in this way works well when the patient's arms are too weak to use for upper trunk exercise. This combination is also useful when the patient has pain in the neck or upper trunk. The pivot of emphasis can be changed to trunk lateral flexion. See Sect. 10.3.3.

Alternative Positions

Use this lower extremity combination on the mats to facilitate rolling from side-lying or prone to supine.

> **→ Points to remember**
> - **Resistance with your distal hand to the knee extension controls the trunk activity**
> - **The desired activity is trunk elongation, not lumbar spine hyperextension**

10.3.3 Trunk Lateral Flexion

The lateral flexion pattern can be done with a trunk flexion bias or an extension bias. To exercise the motion, use the bilateral leg flexion or extension patterns with full hip rotation.

Left Lateral Flexion with Flexion Bias

Begin at the shortened range of bilateral lower extremity flexion to the left. You may place the legs here if the patient's condition requires that.

Command

"Swing your feet away from me (to the left)." If you are working with straight leg patterns, a good command is: "Turn your heels away from me."

Resistance

With your proximal hand give traction through the thighs to lock in the hip flexion. Lateral pressure resists the lateral hip motion. With your distal hand lock in the knees and feet and resist the hip rotation.

Movement

The hips and knees are flexed to the left. As the hips rotate left past the groove of the flexion pattern, the lumbar spine side-bends to the left and the pelvis moves up toward the ribs.

→ **Points to remember**
- **Traction through the femurs locks in the trunk flexor muscles**
- **It is the hip rotation that controls the trunk side bend**

Right Lateral Flexion with Extension Bias (Fig. 10.6)

We can exercise this motion in the lengthened or the shortened range of the leg patterns.

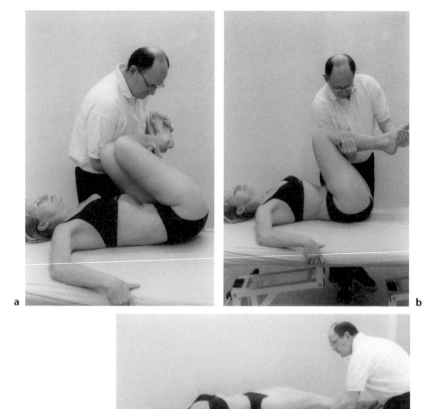

a   b

c

Fig. 10.6. Right lateral flexion with extension bias. **a,b** Lateral flexion in the lengthened range. Resistance to bilateral asymmetrical leg extension: motion of the rotatory component results in the trunk lateral flexion. **c** Lateral flexion in the shortened range

In the Lengthened Range

Begin with the patient's legs in full flexion to the left (the lengthened range of bilateral lower extremity extension to the right) (Fig. 10.6a).

Body Mechanics

Stand in a stride position by the patient's left shoulder. Use your body weight to resist the leg and trunk motion.

Command

"Swing your feet to the right and push your legs away." If you wish, ask for a static rather than a dynamic contraction of the hip and knee extension (Fig. 10.6 b).

Resistance

With your proximal hand resist the hip extension and lateral motion. Your distal hand locks in the knee and foot motion and resists the dynamic hip rotation.

Motion

The hips rotate fully to the right. The lumbar spine extends and side-bends right.

Note: **Allow a few degrees of hip and knee extension to the right.**

In the Shortened Range
You may begin with the patient's legs in full flexion to the left or pre-position the legs in full extension to the right.

Body Mechanics

Stand on the right and use your body as you did for the pattern of trunk extension to the right.

Command

"Kick and turn your heels toward me." "Keep your legs down and turn your heels to me again."

Resistance

Give the same resistance as you did for trunk extension. Allow full hip rotation.

Motion

The patient's legs extend to the right with full hip rotation. The lumbar spine extends and side-bends right (Fig. 10.6 c).

→ **Points to remember**
- **In the lengthened range traction through the femurs locks in the trunk extensor muscles**
- **It is the hip rotation that controls the trunk side bend**

10.4 Combining Patterns for the Trunk

You can combine the upper and lower trunk patterns to suit the needs of the patient. When treating an adult patient work in positions where you can handle the patterns comfortably. You may pre-position the patient's arms and legs in the shortened range of the patterns you are exercising. Choose techniques suited to the patient's needs and strengths. Some trunk combinations are:

- Upper and lower trunk flexion:
  ▶ With counter-rotation of the trunk
    Chopping to the left with bilateral leg flexion to the right (Fig. 10.7)

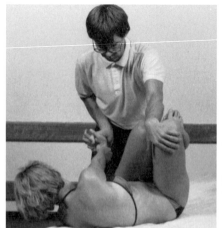
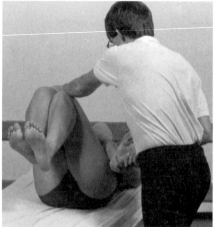
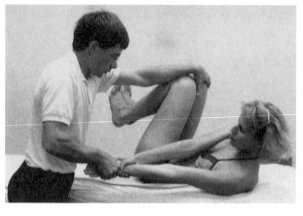

Fig. 10.7 a–c. Trunk combination: chopping to the left with bilateral leg flexion to the right

- Upper trunk flexion with lower trunk extension:
  - ▶ With trunk counter-rotation
    Chopping to the left with bilateral leg extension to the right
  - ▶ Without trunk counter-rotation
    Chopping to the left with bilateral leg extension to the left
- Upper and lower trunk extension:
  - ▶ With counter-rotation of the trunk
    Lifting to the right with bilateral leg extension to the left. Use a static contraction of the lower extremity extension pattern from the flexed position (Fig. 10.8).
  - ▶ Without counter-rotation of the trunk
    Lifting to the left with bilateral leg extension to the left

! Note: Use static contractions of the lower extremity extension pattern from the flexed position.

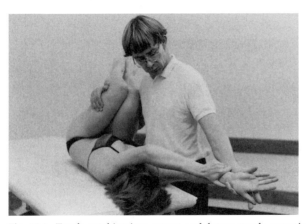

Fig. 10.8. Trunk combination: upper and lower trunk extension using lifting to the right and bilateral leg extension to the left

- Upper trunk extension with lower trunk flexion:
  - ▶ With trunk counter-rotation
    Lifting to the left with bilateral leg flexion to the right
  - ▶ Without trunk counter-rotation
    Lifting to the left with bilateral leg flexion to the left (Fig. 10.9)

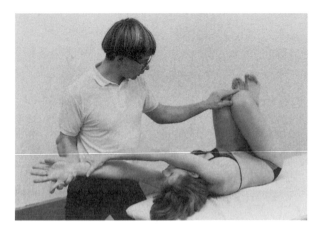

Fig. 10.9. Trunk combination: lifting to the left with bilateral leg flexion to the left

References

Angel RW, Eppler WG Jr (1967) Synergy of contralateral muscles in normal subjects and patients with neurologic disease. Arch Phys Med Rehabil 48:233–239
Kendall FP, McCreary EK (1983) Muscles, testing and function. Williams and Wilkins, Baltimore

11 Mat Activities

11.1 Introduction: Why Do Mat Activities?

The mat program involves the patient in activities incorporating both movement and stability. They range from single movements, such as unilateral scapula motions, to complex combinations requiring both stabilization and motion, such as crawling or knee walking. The activities are done in different positions, for function and to vary the effects of reflexes or gravity. The therapist also chooses positions that can help control abnormal or undesired movements. Mat treatment unites all the parts of the PNF philosophy. In this situation it is easy to begin with activities that are strong and pain free and work toward improving those functions that need improvement. Because the mat activities involve many parts of the body, irradiation from the strong parts is easier to achieve. Last (but not least) the work can be fun.

When working with an infant, it may be necessary to progress treatment using activities that suit the developmental level of the individual. With the adult patient more mature or advanced activities can be used before the more basic activities. The therapist must keep in mind the changing ways in which we accomplish physical tasks as we age (Van Sant 1991).

Functional goals direct the choice of mat activities. An activity, such as getting from supine to sitting, is broken down and the parts practiced. As there are many different ways in which a person can accomplish any activity, treatments should include a variety of movements. For example, to increase trunk and leg strength, the patient may begin treatment with resisted exercises in sitting and side-sitting. The treatment then progresses to positions involving more extremity weight bearing. As the patient's abilities increase, exercises that combine balance and motion in bridging, quadruped, and kneeling positions are used. With all functional activities, the patient learns:
1. *Mobility:* moving into a position
2. *Stability:* stabilizing (balance) in that position

Depending on the patient's condition, you may start the activities with stability or mobility. For example, a patient with quadriplegia may need to practice stability in the sitting position before working on getting to sitting (mobility).

3. *Skill:* combining functional motion with stability or while moving from one position to another.

In every new position we can emphasize one or more of these aspects of motor control, depending on our treatment goals. To reach these goals we use the PNF basic procedures and techniques.

Once patients achieve a reasonable degree of competence in an activity they can safely practice on the mats alone or with minimal supervision. Learning and practicing the skills necessary for self-care and gait is easier for the patients when they feel secure and comfortable.

11.2 Treatment Goals

THERAPEUTIC GOALS ▬▬▬▬▬▬▬▬▬▬▬▬▬▬▬▬▬▬▬▬
We can accomplish many functional treatment goals with mat activities:
▶ Teaching and practicing functional activity such as rolling and moving from one position to another
▶ Training stability in different positions
▶ Increasing coordination
▶ Strengthening functional activities
▶ Gaining mobility in joints and muscles
▶ Normalizing tone

11.3 Basic Procedures

The therapist should employ all the basic procedures to heighten the patient's capacity to work effectively and with minimum fatigue. **Approximation** promotes stabilization and balance. **Traction** and **stretch** (stimulus or reflex) increase the patient's ability to move. Use of correct **grips** and proper **body position** enables the therapist to guide the patient's motion. **Resistance** enhances and reinforces the learning of an activity. Properly graded resistance strengthens the weaker motions. Resisting strong motions provides irradiation into the weaker motions or muscles. **Timing for emphasis** enables the therapist to use strong motions to exercise the weaker ones. Use **patterns** when appropriate to improve performance of functional activities. **Commands** should be clear and relate to the functional goal: stabilization or motion.

11.4 Techniques

All the techniques are suitable for use with mat activities:
▶ To emphasize *Stability* use: Stabilizing Reversal, Rhythmic Stabilization

▶ To emphasize *Mobility* use: Combination of Isotonics, Rhythmic Initiation, Dynamic Reversals, Repeated Stretch
▶ To emphasize *Skill* use a combination of moving and stabilizing techniques. For example, Stabilizing Reversals to stabilize the trunk in sitting combined with Combination of Isotonics for controlled functional arm activity.

11.5 Mat Activities

In mat treatments, we can have both prone and supine activities, but there is much duplication of positions and activities. When necessary teach the patient to stabilize in each new position.

The following examples of mat activities and exercises are not an all-inclusive list but are samples only. As you work with your patients you will find many other positions and actions to help them achieve their functional goals.

Table 11.1

Prone activities	Supine activities
Roll from supine to prone	Roll from prone to supine
Roll from prone to side-lying	Roll from supine to side-lying
Prone on elbows	From supine to side-sitting
Prone on hands	Scooting in side-sitting
Quadruped	From side-sitting to quadruped
Side-sitting	From side-sitting to long-sitting
Sit on heels	Scooting in long-sitting
Kneeling	Short-sitting (legs over edge of mats)
Half-kneeling	Scooting in short-sitting
Hands-and-feet (arched position)	Get to standing
Get to standing	

11.5.1 Rolling

Certain functional activities such as rolling normally have some concentric and some eccentric components.

If the therapist wants to facilitate rolling from the supine into the prone position, the first part of the activity is a concentric action of the flexor chain (trunk flexors, neck flexors and hip flexors) (Fig. 11.2 a, b). When the patient rolls from the mid-position (Fig. 11.3 b) into the prone position, we see an eccentric activity of the extensor chain (trunk extensors, neck extensors and hip extensors). To facilitate this eccentric activity we should move our hands to the ischial tuberosity and posterior on the top of the shoulder to resist the extensor chain. We ask the patient to let us push him forward, but slowly.

Rolling is both a functional activity and an exercise for the entire body. The therapist can learn a great deal about patients by watching them roll. Some people roll using flexion movements, others use extension, and others push with an arm or a leg. Some find it more difficult to roll in one direction than in the other, or from one starting position. The ideal is for individuals to adjust to any condition placed upon them and still be able to roll easily.

THERAPEUTIC GOALS ▆▆▆▆▆▆▆▆▆▆▆▆▆▆▆▆▆▆▆▆▆▆▆▆▆▆▆▆▆▆▆▆▆

The goal of rolling can be:
▶ Strengthening of trunk muscles
▶ Increasing the patient's ability to roll
▶ Mobilizing the trunk, scapula, shoulder or hip
▶ Normalizing the muscle tone etc.

The therapist uses whatever combination of scapula, pelvis, neck or extremity motions best facilitates and reinforces the desired motions.

Scapula

Resistance to either of the anterior scapular patterns facilitates forward rolling. Resisting the posterior scapular patterns facilitates rolling back. Use the appropriate grips for the chosen scapular pattern. To get increased facilitation, tell the patient to move the head in the same direction as the scapula.

The command given can be an explicit direction or a simple action command. An explicit direction for rolling using scapular anterior depression would be "pull your shoulder down toward your opposite hip, lift your head, and roll forward." A simple action command for the same motion is "pull down." A simple command for rolling back using posterior elevation is "push back" or "shrug." Telling the patient to look in the direction of the scapula motion is a good command for the head movement.

To start, place the scapula in the elongated range to stretch the scapular muscles. To stretch the trunk muscles, continue moving the scapula farther in the same diagonal until the trunk muscles are elongated. Resist the initial contraction at the scapula enough to hold back on the scapular motion until you feel or see the patient's trunk muscles contract. When the trunk muscles begin to contract, allow both the scapula and trunk to move. You can lock in the scapula at the end of its range of motion by giving more resistance and either traction or approximation. Now exercise the trunk muscles and the rolling motion with repeated contractions for the trunk muscles.

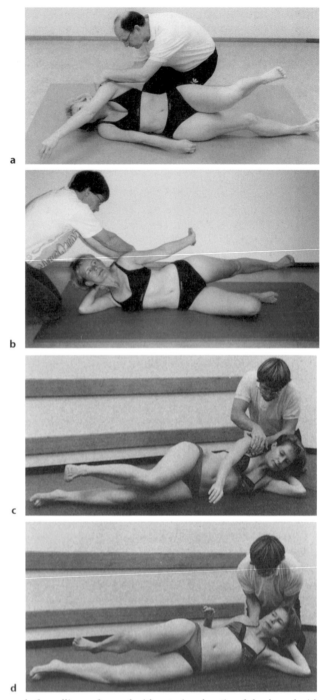

Fig. 11.1 a–d. Using the scapula for rolling: **a** forward with anterior elevation; **b** backward with posterior depression; **c** forward with anterior depression; **d** backward with posterior elevation

Anterior Elevation

Roll forward with trunk rotation and extension. Facilitate with neck extension and rotation in the direction of the rolling motion (Fig. 11.1 a).

Posterior Depression

Roll back with trunk extension, lateral flexion, and rotation. Facilitate with neck lateral flexion and full rotation in the direction of the rolling motion (Fig. 11.1 b).

Anterior Depression

Roll forward with trunk flexion. Facilitate with neck flexion in the direction of the rolling motion (Fig. 11.1 c).

Posterior Elevation

Roll back with trunk extension. Facilitate with neck extension in the direction of the rolling motion (Fig. 11.1 d).

Pelvis

Resistance to pelvic anterior patterns facilitates rolling forward, resisting posterior patterns facilitates rolling back. Use the appropriate grips for the chosen pattern. Ask for neck flexion to reinforce rolling forward, extension for rolling back.

The commands for pelvic motion are similar to those for the scapula. For rolling forward using anterior elevation the explicit command would be "pull your pelvis up and roll forward". The simple command for the same motion is "pull." For rolling back using posterior depression a specific command would be "sit down into my hand and roll back." The simple command for that action is "push." Facilitate with the appropriate neck motion.

To start, place the pelvis in its elongated range. To stretch the trunk further, continue moving the pelvis in the same diagonal until the trunk is completely elongated. Resist the initial contraction at the pelvis until you feel or see all of the desired trunk muscles contract. Then allow both the pelvis and trunk to move. You can lock in the pelvis at the end of its range of motion by giving more resistance and by giving traction or approximation. Then exercise the rolling motion with repeated contractions for the trunk muscles.

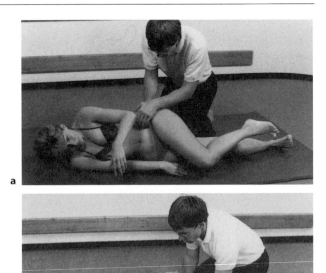

Fig. 11.2 a, b. Using the pelvis for rolling: **a** forward with anterior elevation; **b** backward with posterior depression

Anterior Elevation

Roll forward with trunk flexion, facilitate with neck flexion (Fig. 11.2 a).

Posterior Depression

Roll back with trunk extension, facilitate with neck extension (Fig. 11.2 b).

Posterior Elevation

Roll back with lateral shortening of the trunk, facilitate with neck rotation to the same side.

Anterior Depression

Roll forward with trunk extension and rotation, facilitate with neck extension and rotation into that direction.

→ **Points to remember**
- **Rolling is the activity, the scapula and pelvis are the handle**
- **The rolling should occur because of facilitation from the scapula or pelvis**

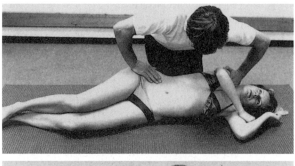

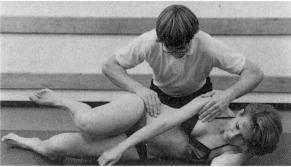

Fig. 11.3a,b. Rolling forward with pelvic anterior elevation and scapular anterior depression

Scapula and Pelvis

A combination for rolling forward: the pelvis in anterior elevation, the scapula in anterior depression (Fig. 11.3).

A combination for rolling backward: the pelvis in posterior depression, the scapula in posterior elevation (Fig. 11.4).

Upper Extremities

When the patient has a strong arm, combine it with the scapula to strengthen the trunk muscles and to facilitate rolling in the same way as with the scapula alone. Adduction (anterior) patterns facilitate rolling forward. Abduction (posterior) patterns facilitate rolling back. The elbow may flex, extend or remain in one position during the activity. Resist the strongest elbow muscles for irradiation into the trunk muscles. The patient's head should move with the arm.

Your distal grip is on the hand or distal forearm and can control the entire extremity. Your proximal grip can vary: a grip on or near the scapula is often the most effective. Your proximal hand can also be used to guide and resist the patient's head motion.

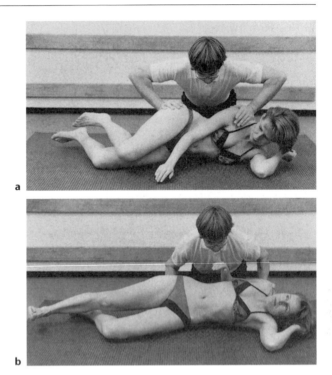

Fig. 11.4a,b. Rolling backward with pelvic posterior depression and scapular posterior elevation

The commands you use can be specific or simple. For rolling forward using the pattern of extension–adduction the specific command may be "squeeze my hand and pull your arm down to your opposite hip. Lift your head, and roll." A simple command would be "squeeze and pull, lift your head." For rolling back using the pattern of flexion–abduction the specific command might be "wrist back, lift your arm up and follow your hand with your eyes. Roll back." The simple command would be "lift your arm up and look at your hand."

Take the patient's arm into the elongated range and traction to stretch the arm and scapular muscles. Further elongation with traction will elongate or stretch the synergistic trunk muscles. Hold back on the initial arm motion until you feel or see the patient's trunk muscles contract, then allow the arm and trunk to move. You can lock in the patient's arm at any strong point in its range of motion, then exercise the trunk muscles and the rolling motion with repeated contractions. *The exercise is for the trunk muscles and not for the shoulder muscles (change the pivot).* Approximation through the arm with resistance to rotation works well to lock in the arm toward the end of its range.

Using one arm

▶ Rolling forward with trunk-extension, lateral flexion and rotation.
Facilitate with neck extension and rotation in the direction of the rolling.
  • Patterns: Flexion–adduction–external rotation (Fig. 11.5 a). Ulnar thrust
    pattern.
▶ Rolling back with trunk extension, lateral flexion, and rotation. Facilitate
with neck lateral flexion and full rotation in the direction of the rolling
motion.
  • Patterns: Extension–abduction–internal rotation (Fig. 11.5 b). Ulnar
    withdrawal pattern.

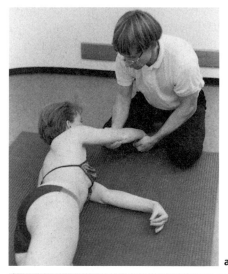

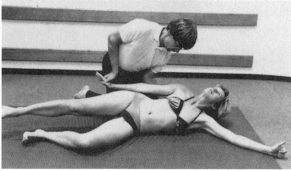

Fig. 11.5. Using one arm for rolling: **a** forward with flexion–adduction; **b** backward with
extension–abduction

▶ Rolling forward with trunk flexion. Facilitate with neck flexion in the direction of the rolling motion.
  • Patterns: Extension–adduction–internal rotation (Fig. 11.5 c, d). Radial thrust pattern
▶ Rolling back with trunk extension. Facilitate with neck extension in the direction of the rolling motion.
  • Pattern: Flexion–abduction (Fig. 11.5 e, f).

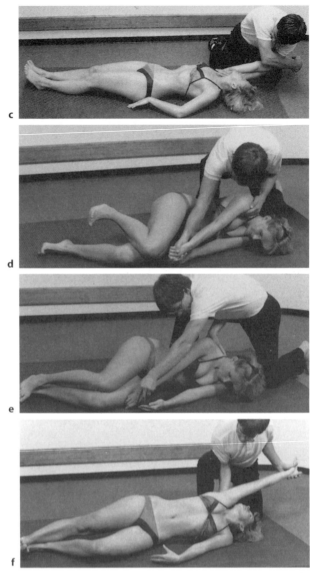

Fig. 11.5 d–f. Using one arm for rolling: c, d forward with extension–adduction; e, f backward with flexion–abduction

Using Bilateral Combinations

▶ Rolling forward with trunk flexion: Chopping (Fig. 11.6 a) and Reverse of Chopping (Fig. 11.6 b)
▶ Rolling back with trunk extension: Lifting (Fig. 11.6 c, d)

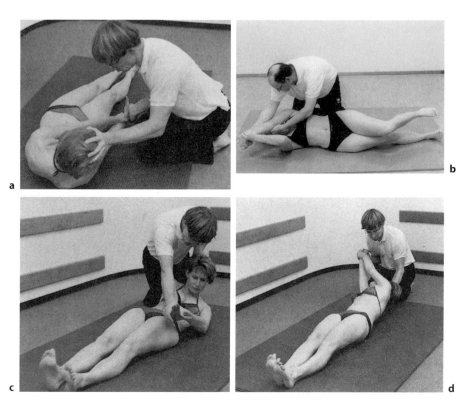

Fig. 11.6. Using both arms for rolling: **a** forward with chopping; **b** forward with reversal of chopping; **c, d** backward with lifting

---

→ **Points to remember**
● **Rolling is the activity, the arm is the handle**
● **The techniques are applied to the trunk for the rolling motion**

Lower Extremities

Use the patient's leg to facilitate rolling and to strengthen trunk muscles in the same way as with the arm. The knee may flex, extend or remain in one position. As with the elbow, resist the strongest knee muscles to facilitate the rolling. Flexion (anterior) patterns facilitate rolling forward, extension (posterior) patterns facilitate rolling back. The patient's head will facilitate rolling forward by going into flexion, and rolling back by going into extension.

Your distal grip is on the foot and can control the entire extremity. To make the activity effective give the principal resistance to the knee activity rather than the hip. Your proximal grip may be on the thigh or pelvis. When the pattern of flexion–abduction is used you may put your proximal hand on the opposite iliac crest to facilitate trunk flexion.

The commands can be specific or simple. A specific command for rolling forward using flexion-abduction is "foot up, pull your leg up and out and roll away." A simple command is "pull your leg up." For rolling back using the pattern of extension–adduction the specific command is "push your foot down, kick your leg back, and roll back toward me." A simple command may be "kick back."

Bring the patient's leg into the elongated range of the pattern using traction to stretch the muscles of the extremity and lower trunk. Hold back on the leg motion until you see or feel the patient's trunk muscles contract then allow the leg and trunk to move. Lock in the leg at any strong point in its range of motion and exercise the trunk muscles and the rolling motion with repeated contractions.

→ **Points to remember**
- **Rolling is the activity, the leg is the handle**
- **The techniques are applied to the trunk for the rolling motion**

Using One Leg

▶ Flexion–adduction (Fig. 11.7 a, b): Rolling forward with trunk flexion
▶ Extension–abduction (Fig. 11.7 c, d): Rolling back with trunk extension and elongation
▶ Flexion–abduction (Fig. 11.7 e): Rolling forward with trunk lateral flexion, flexion, and rotation
▶ Extension–adduction (Fig. 11.7 f): Rolling back with trunk extension, elongation, and rotation

Bilateral Combinations

▶ Lower extremity flexion (Fig. 11.8 a): Rolling forward with trunk flexion
▶ Lower extremity extension (Fig. 11.8 b): Rolling back with trunk extension

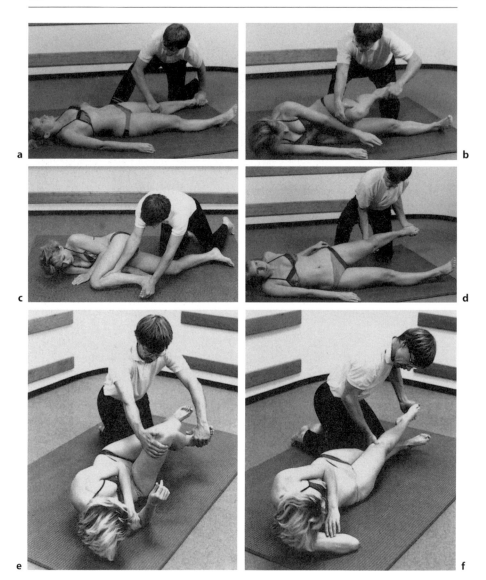

Fig. 11.7 a–f. Using one leg for rolling: **a, b** forward with flexion–adduction; **c, d** backward with extension–abduction; **e** forward with flexion–abduction; **f** backward with extension–adduction

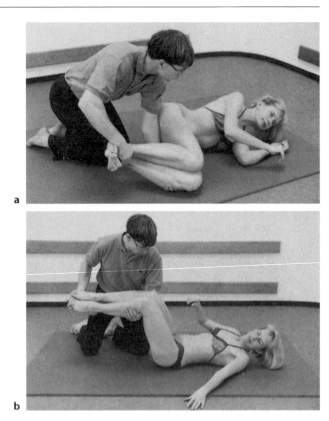

Fig. 11.8 a, b. Using both legs for rolling: **a** forward with flexion; **b** backward with extension

Neck Patterns (see Fig. 9.8)

The head and neck move with the all rolling motions. If the patient does not have pain free or strong motion in the scapula or arm it may be necessary to use the neck alone to facilitate rolling. When using neck flexion the main force is traction, for neck extension use gentle compression.

- Neck flexion: Rolling forward from supine to side-lying (see Fig. 9.8 a, b)
- Neck extension: Rolling backward from side-lying to supine (see Fig. 9.8 c)

> → **Points to remember**
> - **Rolling is the activity, the neck is the handle**
> - **For more sideways motion, allow more neck rotation**
> - **The techniques are applied to the trunk for the rolling motion**

11.5.2 Prone on Elbows (Forearm Support)

Lying prone on the elbows is an ideal position for working on stability of the head, neck, and shoulders. Resisted neck motions can be done effectively and without pain in this position. Resisted arm motions will strengthen not only the moving arm but also the shoulder and scapular muscles of the weight-bearing arm. The position is also a good one for exercising facial muscles and swallowing.

Assuming the Position

The patient can get to prone on elbows from many positions. We suggest three methods to facilitate the patient who is not able to assume this position independently.
▶ From side-sitting
▶ Rolling over from a supine position
▶ From a prone position (Fig. 11.9 a–d)

Resist the patient's concentric contractions if they move against gravity into the position (e. g., moving from prone to prone on elbows, Fig. 11.9 c, d). Resist eccentric control if the motion is gravity assisted (e. g., moving from side-sitting to prone on elbows).

Stabilizing

When the patient is secure in the position, begin stabilization with approximation through the scapula and resistance in diagonal and rotary directions. It is important that patients maintain their scapulae in a functional position. Do not allow their trunk to sag. With the head and neck aligned with the trunk, give gentle resistance at the head for stabilization (Fig. 11.9 e). Rhythmic Stabilization works well here. Use Stabilizing Reversal with those patients who cannot do isometric contractions.

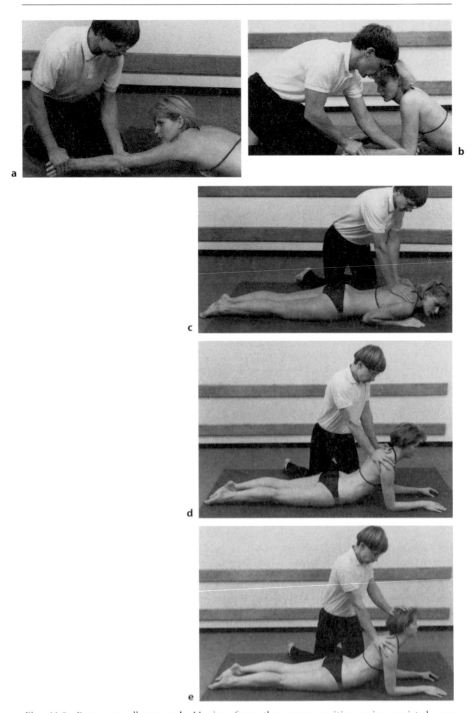

Fig. 11.9. Prone on elbows. **a,b** Moving from the prone position using resisted arm patterns. **c,d** moving from the prone position with facilitation of the scapula; **e** stabilization

Motion

With the patient prone on elbows you can exercise the head, neck, upper trunk, and arms. A few exercises are described here but let your imagination help you discover others.

▶ Head and neck motion: resist flexion, extension, and rotation. Try Slow Reversals and Combination of Isotonics.

▶ Upper trunk rotation: combine this motion with head and neck rotation. Use Slow Reversals and resist at the scapula or scapula and head (Fig. 11.10 a, b).

▶ Weight shift: shift weight completely to one arm. Combine the techniques Combination of Isotonics and Slow Reversals.

▶ Arm motion: after the weight shift, resist any pattern of the free arm. Use Combination of Isotonics followed by an active reversal to the antagonistic pattern. Use Stabilizing Reversals on the weight-bearing side (Fig. 11.10 c, d).

→ **Points to remember**
- **This is an active position. The patient should not "hang" on the shoulder blades**
- **It the position causes back pain you can put a support under the patient's abdomen**

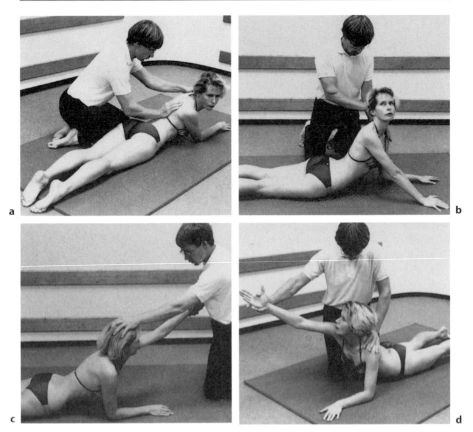

Fig. 11.10a–d. Prone on the elbows: stability and motion. **a** Reciprocal scapular patterns; **b** resistance to head and scapula; **c** resistance to head and raised arm; **d** resistance to raised arm and contralateral scapula

11.5.3 Side-Sitting

This is an intermediate position between lying down and sitting. There is weight-bearing through the arm, leg, and trunk on one side. The other arm can be used for support or for functional activities. For function the patient should learn mobility in this position (scooting).

Side-sitting is a good position for exercising the scapular and pelvic patterns. Movement in reciprocal scapular and pelvic combinations promotes trunk mobility. Stabilizing contractions of the reciprocal patterns promote trunk stability.

We list below some of the usual activities. Do not restrict yourself only to those given; let your imagination guide you.
▶ Assuming the position
  • From side-lying
  • From prone on elbows (Fig. 11.11)
  • From sitting
  • From the quadruped position
▶ Balancing
  • Scapula and pelvic *motions* (Fig. 11.12 a–d)
  • Upper extremity weight bearing (Fig. 11.12 e)
▶ Leg patterns (Fig. 11.12 f)
▶ Scooting (Fig. 11.12 g, h)
▶ Moving to sitting
▶ Moving to prone on elbows
▶ Moving to the quadruped position

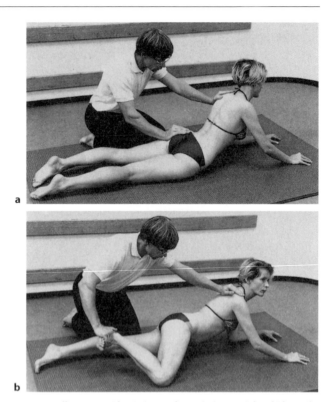

Fig. 11.11. Moving from prone on elbows to side-sitting. a,b Resisting weight shift to the left

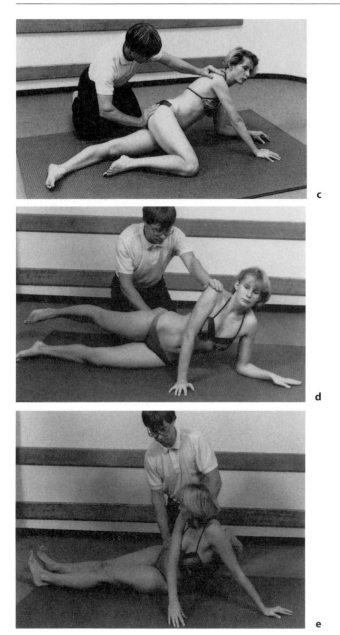

c

d

e

Fig. 11.11. Moving from prone on elbows to side-sitting. c–e Resistance at scapula and pelvis

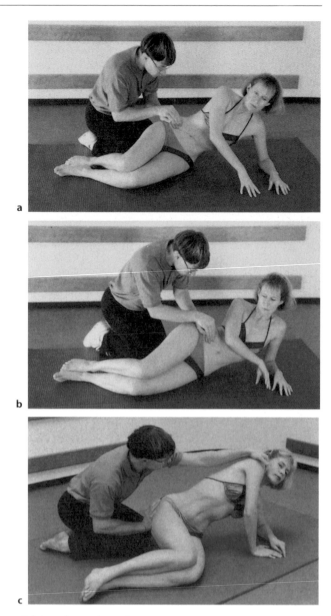

Fig. 11.12. Side-sitting. a–c Pelvis and scapula motion

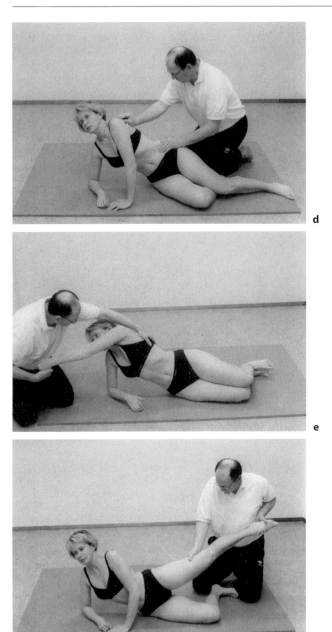

d

e

f

Fig. 11.12. Side-sitting. **d** emphasis on weight-bearing activity on the right shoulder; **e** resistance to the left arm flexion–adduction and resistance for elongation of the left side of the trunk; **f** hip extension–abduction

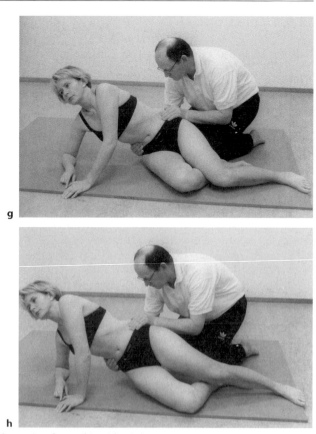

Fig. 11.12. Side-sitting. **g, h** Moving forward in side-sitting

11.5.4 Quadruped

In the quadruped position patients can exercise their trunk, hips, knees, and shoulders. The ability to move on the floor is a functional reason for activity in this position. The patient can move to a piece of furniture or to another room.

Be sure that the scapular muscles are strong enough to support the weight of the upper trunk. There must be no knee pain. Because the spine is in a non-weight-bearing position, when spinal pain or stabilization is the problem working in this position will make many activities possible.

Use the techniques Stabilizing Reversals and Rhythmic Stabilization to gain stability in the trunk and extremity joints. Resist rocking motions in all directions using Combination of Isotonics, Dynamic Reversals (Slow Reversals) and a combination of these techniques to exercise the extremities with weight bearing. Resisted crawling enhances the patient's ability to combine motion with stability.

When the patient is assuming and working in the quadruped position the therapist gives resistance at scapula or pelvis, at the head and a combination of these areas.

▶ Assuming the position
   • From prone on elbows (Fig. 11.13 a–e)
   • From side-sitting (Fig. 11.13 f, g)
▶ Balancing (Fig. 11.14)
▶ Trunk exercise (Fig. 11.15)
▶ Rocking forward and back (Fig. 11.16)
▶ Arm and leg exercises (Fig. 11.17)
▶ Crawling: in addition to giving resistance to the scapula, pelvis and neck the therapist also gives resistance
   • to leg motions (Fig. 11.18)
   • to arm motions

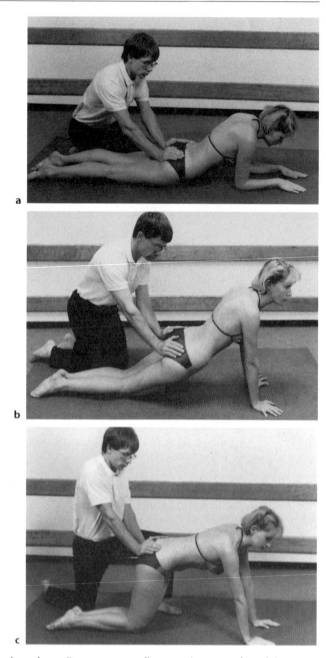

Fig. 11.13. Moving to quadruped. a–c From prone on elbows, resistance at the pelvis

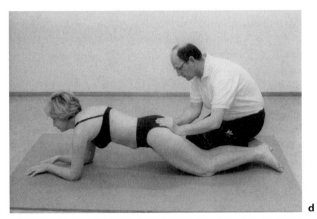

d

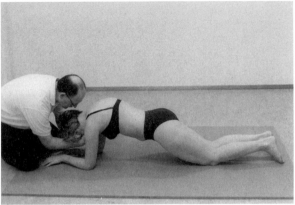

e

Fig. 11.13. Moving to quadruped. **d** From prone on elbows, mid-position, resistance to the pelvis; **e** resistance to neck flexion

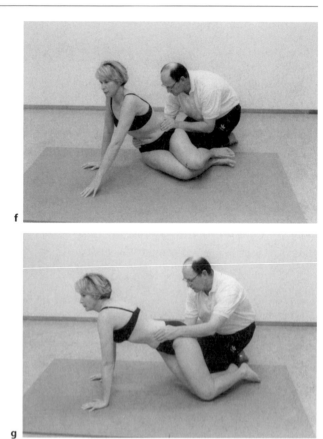

Fig. 11.13. Moving to quadruped. f, g Moving from side-sitting resistance at pelvis

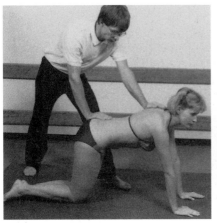 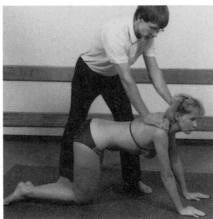

a   **b**

Fig. 11.14 a, b. Balancing in quadruped

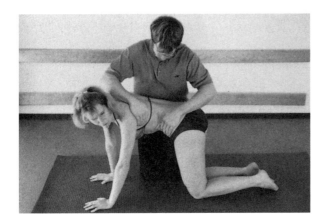

Fig. 11.15. Quadruped, trunk lateral flexion

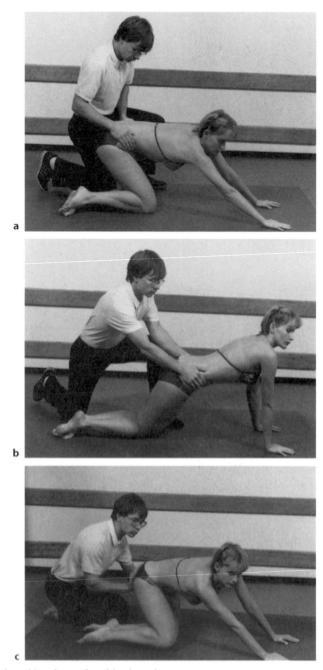

Fig. 11.16a–c. Quadruped, rocking forward and backward

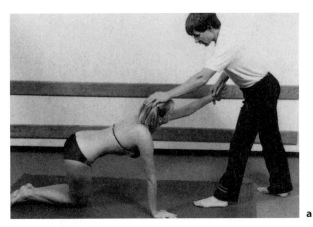

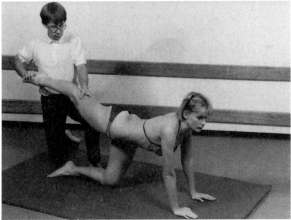

Fig. 11.17 a, b. Quadruped, arm and leg exercise

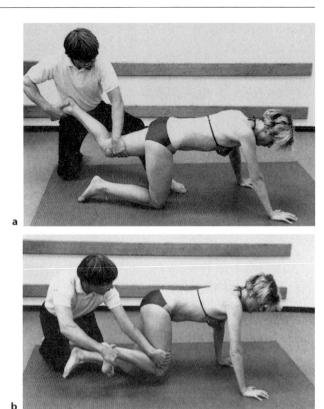

Fig. 11.18 a, b. Crawling, resisting leg motions

11.5.5 Kneeling

In a kneeling position patients exercise their trunk, hips and knees, while the arms are free or used for support. For function patients go from the kneeling position to standing, or move on the floor to a piece of furniture such as a bed or sofa. If the patient is unable to work in kneeling, for example because of knee pain, most of the kneeling activities can be done in the kneeling down (sitting on the feet) position.

To increase trunk strength and stability resist at the scapula and pelvis using Stabilizing Reversals or Rhythmic Stabilization. To increase the strength, coordination, and range of motion of the hips and knees exercise the patient moving between kneeling and a side-sitting position. Combination of Isotonics will exercise the concentric and eccentric muscular functions.

▶ Assuming the position
  • From a side-sitting position (Fig. 11.19a,b) or a kneeling-down (sitting on your feet) (Fig. 11.19c–f)
  • From a quadruped position (Fig. 11.20)

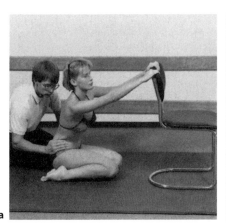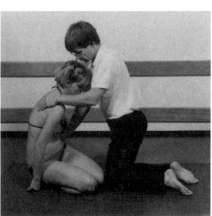

a   b

Fig. 11.19. Assuming the kneeling position. **a, b** Moving from side-sitting to kneeling

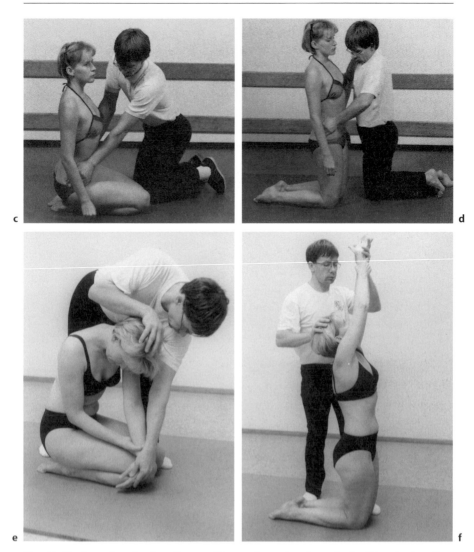

Fig. 11.19. Assuming the kneeling position. **c,d** moving from heel sitting to kneeling, resistance at pelvis; **e,f** resisted lifting to the left

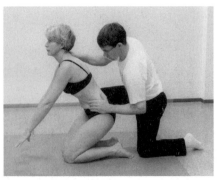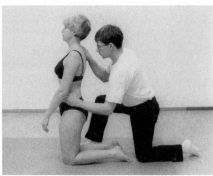

a   b

Fig. 11.20 a, b. Moving from quadruped to kneeling

▶ Balancing
  • Resistance at the scapula and head (Fig. 11.21 a, b)
  • Resistance at the pelvis
  • Resistance at pelvis and scapula (Fig. 11.21 c)
  • Resistance at the trunk and head (Fig. 11.21 d)
  • Resistance to the arms sitting on your heels (Fig. 11.21 e, f)
▶ Walking on the knees
  • Forward (Fig. 11.22 a, b)
  • Backward (Fig. 11.22 c)
  • Sideways (Fig. 11.22 d, e)

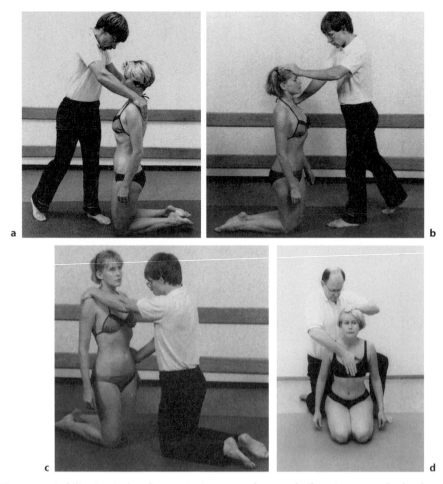

Fig. 11.21. Stabilization in kneeling. **a** Resistance at the scapula; **b** resistance at the head and scapula; **c** resistance at the pelvis and scapula; **d** resistance to the sternum and head

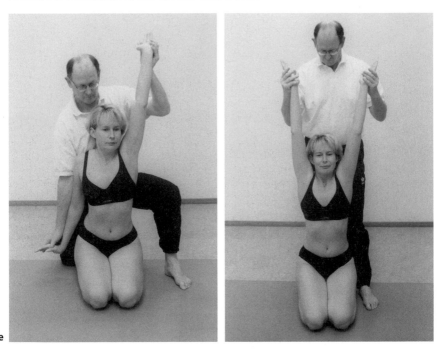

e   f

Fig. 11.21. Stabilization in sitting on your heels. **e** bilateral asymmetrical arm patterns; **f** bilateral symmetrical arm patterns

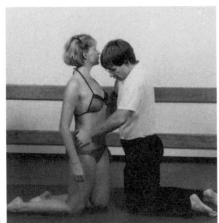

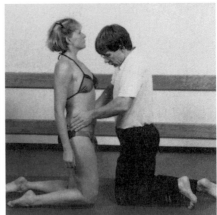

a   b

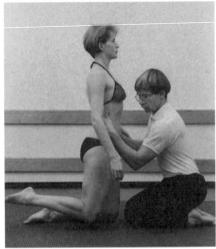

Fig. 11.22 a-e. Walking on the knees:
a, b forward; c backward; d, e sideways

c

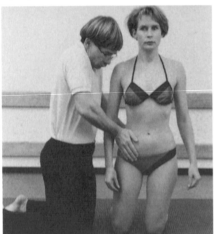

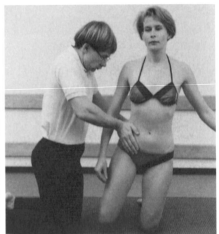

d   e

11.5.6 Half-Kneeling

This is the last position in the kneeling to standing sequence. To complete the work in this position the patients should assume it with either leg forward. Moving from kneeling to half-kneeling requires the patient to shift weight from two to one leg and move the non-weighted leg while maintaining balance. This activity challenges the patient's balance, coordination, range of motion and strength. Use both stabilizing and moving techniques to strengthen trunk and lower extremity muscles. Shifting the weight forward over the front foot promotes an increase in ankle dorsiflexion range.

▶ Assuming the position
  • From a kneeling position (Fig. 11.23)
  • From standing
▶ Balancing (Fig. 11.24 a–c)
▶ Weight shift over back leg with trunk elongation (Fig. 11.24 c)
▶ Weight shift to front leg
▶ Standing up (Fig. 11.25)

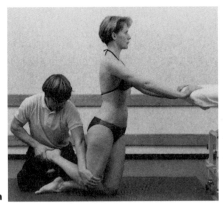
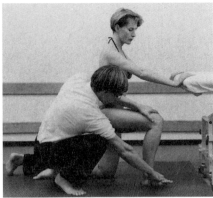

Fig. 11.23 a, b. Moving from kneeling to half-kneeling

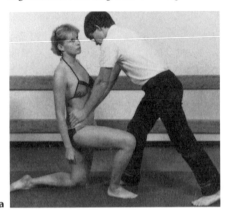
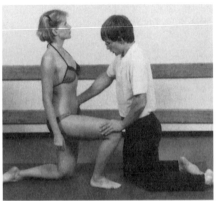

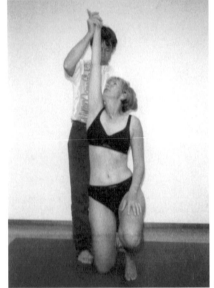

Fig. 11.24 a–c. Balancing and weight shift in half-kneeling. **a** Resistance at the pelvis; **b** resistance at pelvis and forward leg; **c** resistance at arm and head for trunk elongation

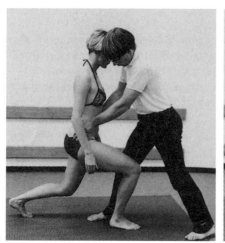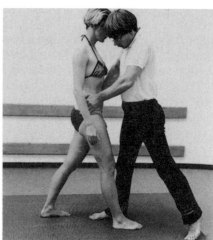

a   b

Fig. 11.25 a, b. Standing up from half-kneeling

11.5.7 From Hands-and-Feet Position (Arched Position on All Fours) to Standing Position and back to Hands-and-Feet Position (Fig. 11.26)

The people who use this activity for function are most often those whose knees are maintained in extension. For example, patients wearing bilateral long leg braces (KAFOs) or those with bilateral above-knee prostheses can go from standing to the floor or from the floor to standing. Use of this position requires full hamstring muscle length.

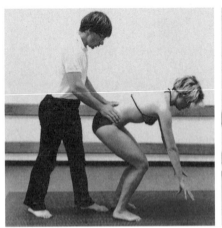
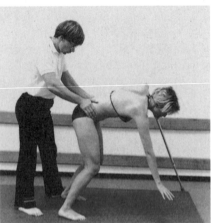

a

b

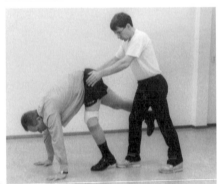

c

Fig. 11.26a-c. Moving to the floor and back up again. a,b Resistance at the pelvis; c guidance at the pelvis, patient with amputation of left leg

11.5.8 Exercise in a Sitting Position

Long-Sitting

This position is functional for bed activities such as eating and dressing. Use all the stabilizing techniques to increase the patient's balance in this position. Because the patient can sit on the floor mats, this is a safe position for independent balance work. Long-sitting is also a good position for exercises to increase arm and trunk strength. All the strengthening exercises are appropriate here. Patients can practice all the lifts used for transfers.

▶ Assuming the position
- From side-sitting
- From supine

▶ Balancing with and without upper extremity support (Fig. 11.27a)
▶ Pushing up exercises
- Resistance at the pelvis and shoulders (Fig. 11.27b–d)
- Resistance at the legs (Fig. 11.27e–h)

▶ Scooting forward (Fig. 11.27i) and backward

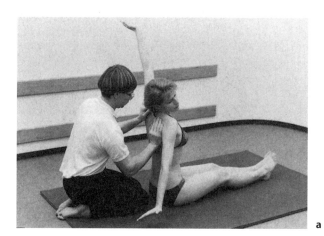

a

Fig. 11.27. Exercises in long-sitting. **a** Stabilization

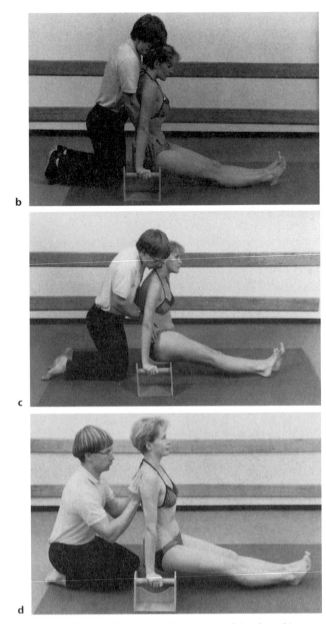

Fig. 11.27. Exercises in long-sitting. b–c pushing up, resistance at pelvis; d pushing up, resistance at scapulae

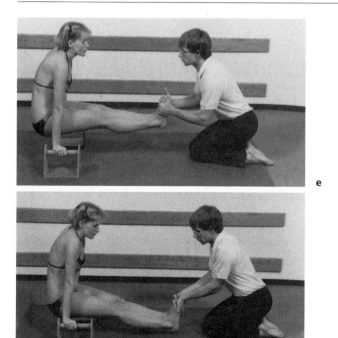

e

f

Fig. 11.27. Exercises in long-sitting. **e, f** pushing up, resistance at the legs

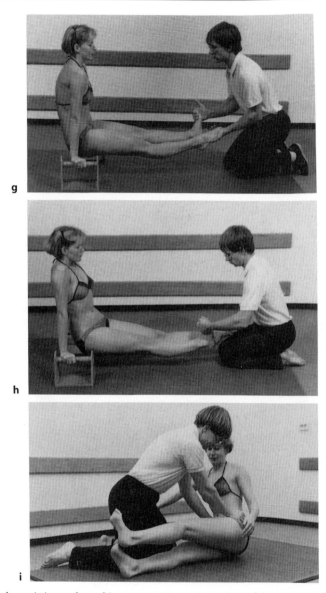

Fig. 11.27. Exercises in long-sitting. **g,h** pushing up, resistance to reciprocal leg patterns; **i** scooting forward

Short-Sitting

To use their arms for other activities, patients need as much trunk control as possible. To reach for distant objects they need to combine trunk stability with trunk, hip, and arm motion. Those patients with spinal problems can learn to stabilize their back while moving at the hip when reaching with their arms.

Patients need to exercise while sitting on the side of the bed and in a chair as well as on the mats. Static exercises in short-sitting will increase the patient's trunk and hip stability. Dynamic exercises will increase trunk and hip motion. Resisting the patient's strong arms will provide irradiation to facilitate weaker trunk and hip muscles. Combining static and dynamic techniques facilitate the patient's ability to combine balance and motion.

▶ Assuming the position from side-lying (Fig. 11.28)
  • Resist the patient's concentric contractions while they move into sitting.
  • Resist the eccentric control as they lie down.

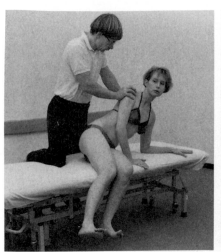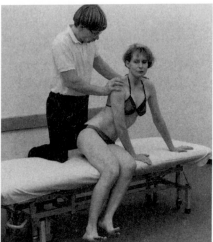

a   b

Fig. 11.28a,b. Moving from side-lying to short-sitting

▶ Balancing
Use Stabilizing Reversals or Rhythmic Stabilization to increase trunk
stability. Resist at the shoulders, pelvis, and head (Fig. 11.29).
  • With and without upper extremity support
  • With and without lower extremity support
▶ Trunk exercises
Use Dynamic Reversals (Slow Reversals) and Combination of Isotonics to
increase the patient's trunk strength and coordination. Resist at the
scapula (Fig. 11.30a,b) or use chopping (Fig. 11.30d) and lifting
combinations to get added irradiation.
  • Trunk flexion (Fig. 11.30c) and extension
  • Reaching forward and to the side with return: this requires hip flexion,
    extension, lateral motion, and rotation with the trunk remaining stable
▶ Moving
These activities teach mobility in sitting and exercise pelvic and hip
muscles.
  • Forward and back (Fig. 11.30e)
  • From side to side

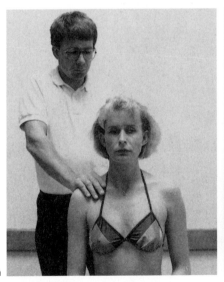
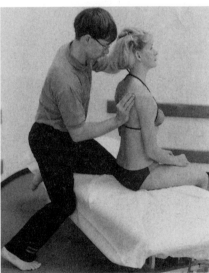

a   b

Fig. 11.29. Stabilization in short-sitting

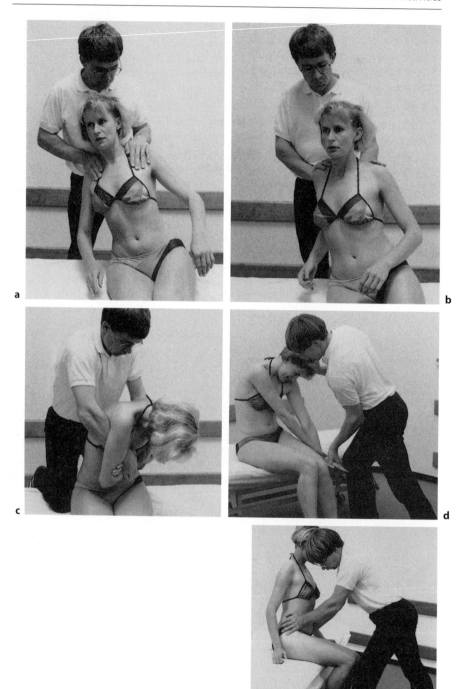

Fig. 11.30. Trunk exercise in short-sitting.
a,b Resistance at scapula; **c** flexion with
traction through arms; **d** chopping;
e moving forward with resistance at pelvis

11.5.9 Bridging

In the hook-lying position the patient exercises with weight-bearing through the feet but without danger of falling. Lifting the pelvis from the supporting surface makes it easier for a person to move and dress in bed.

Working in the hook-lying position requires some selective control of the lower trunk flexors and the leg muscles. Patients must keep their knees flexed while extending their hips and pushing with their feet. When patients push against the mats with their arms, their upper trunk, neck, and upper extremity muscles are exercised. Resist concentric, eccentric, and stabilizing contractions to increase strength and stability in the trunk and lower extremity.

▶ Assuming the hook lying position
   If the patient is unable to assume this position independently:
   • Move from a side-lying position with hips and knees flexed. Facilitate at the knees, pelvis or a combination of these
   • From supine, guide and resist the bilateral pattern of hip flexion with knee flexion
▶ Stabilizing (Fig. 11.31 a)
   • With approximation from the distal femurs into the pelvis combined with stabilizing resistance
   • With approximation from the distal femurs into the feet combined with stabilizing resistance
   • Stabilizing resistance without approximation

Use resistance with approximation at the legs to facilitate lower extremity and trunk stability. Give the resistance in all directions. Resistance in diagonals will recruit more trunk muscle activity. As the patient gains strength, decrease the amount of approximation. Resist the legs together and separately. Resist both legs in the same direction and in opposite directions when working them separately.

▶ Lower trunk rotation in the hook-lying position
The motion begins with the legs moving down diagonally (distally) toward the floor. When the hips have completed their rotation, the pelvis rotates, followed by the spine. The abdominal muscles prevent any increase in lumbar lordosis. The return to upright requires a reverse timing of the motion. The lumbar spine must de-rotate first, then the pelvis, and then the legs. Correct timing of this activity is important. Limit the distance that the legs descend to the ability of the patient to control the motion. Figure 11.31b shows resistance to returning to the upright leg position with lower trunk rotation to the right. You can use Combination of Isotonics and Slow Reversals to teach and strengthen this activity.

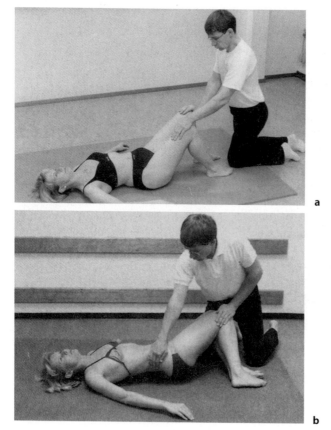

a

b

Fig. 11.31 a, b. Hook lying: **a** stabilization; **b** lower trunk rotation

▶ Bridging
  • Stabilize the pelvis with resistance in all directions (Fig. 11.32a,b, resisting from below; Fig. 11.32c,d resisting from above)
  • Lead with one side of the pelvis
  • Resist static and dynamic rotation of the pelvis
  • Scoot the pelvis from side to side

Use Combination of Isotonics to strengthen the patient's antigravity control.

> **!** Caution: Monitor and control the position of the patient's lumbar spine while the pelvis is elevated.

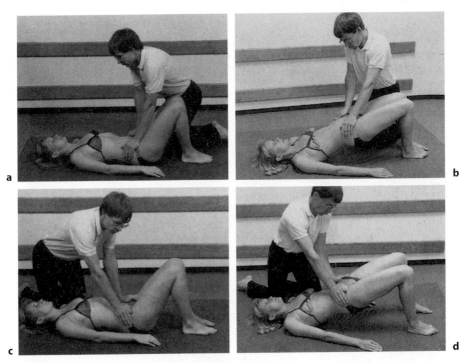

Fig. 11.32a–d. Bridging on two legs in supine position

▶ Other bridging activities
  • Stepping in place
  • Walking the feet: apart, together, to the side, away from the body (into extension) and back
  • Bridge on one leg (Fig. 11.33). The abdominal muscles maintain the pelvis level and the hip muscles on the supporting side work to prevent lateral sway. The more the lifted leg moves into extension or abduction, the harder the supporting muscles must work
  • Bridge while bearing weight on the arms (Figs. 11.34–11.36)

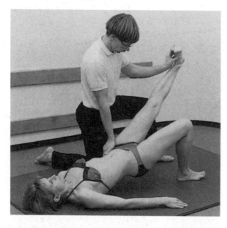

Fig. 11.33. Bridging on one leg

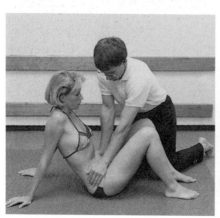

a

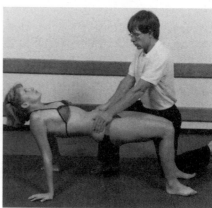

b

Fig. 11.34 a, b. Bridging on the hands

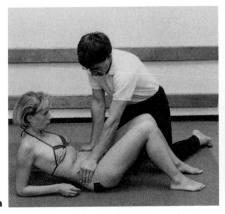
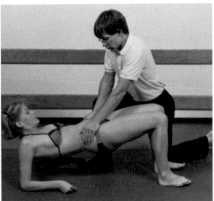

Fig. 11.35 a, b. Bridging on the elbows

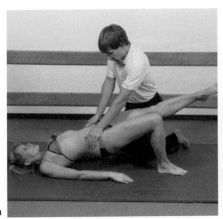
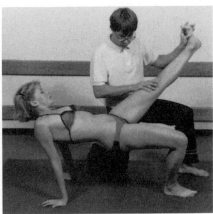

Fig. 11.36. Bridging on the arms and one leg

11.6 Patient Cases in Mat Activities

Patient I   Limited range of motion in the right shoulder (Fig. 11.37)

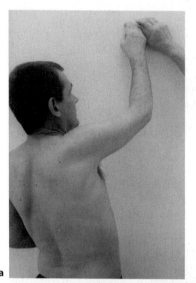

Fig. 11.37. a Demonstrating the limited range of motion in the right shoulder

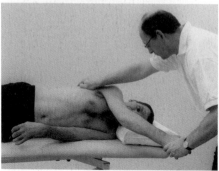

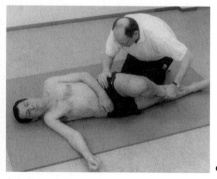

Fig. 11.37. b Contract-relax for the short shoulder extensor and posterior adductor muscles, resistance to the arm pattern of extension–abduction–internal rotation with fixation of the scapula. c Mobilization of the right shoulder using indirect treatment: the lower trunk rolls against a fixed right shoulder

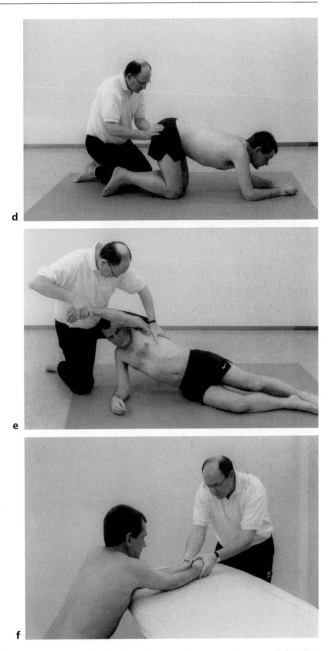

Fig. 11.37. Patient I. Limited range of motion in the right shoulder. **d** Indirect mobilization of the shoulder into flexion by moving the pelvis back and down. **e** Weight-bearing activity of the right shoulder: resistance to the left arm provides irradiation into the involved shoulder. **f** Mobilization of the right shoulder

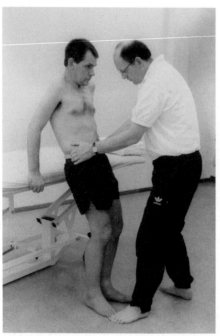

g

Fig. 11.37. Patient I. Limited range of motion in the right shoulder. **g** Strengthening and mobilization of the shoulder in a standing position

Patient II   Incomplete paraplegia in the post-acute phase (Fig. 11.38)

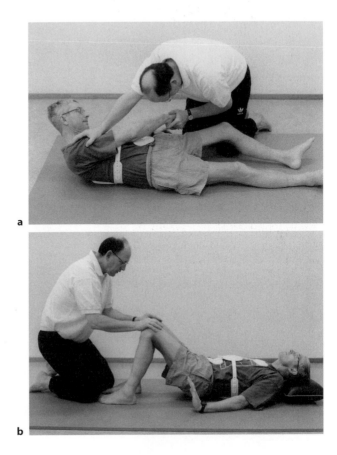

Fig. 11.38. a Rolling: irradiation into lower trunk and hip muscles. **b** Bridging

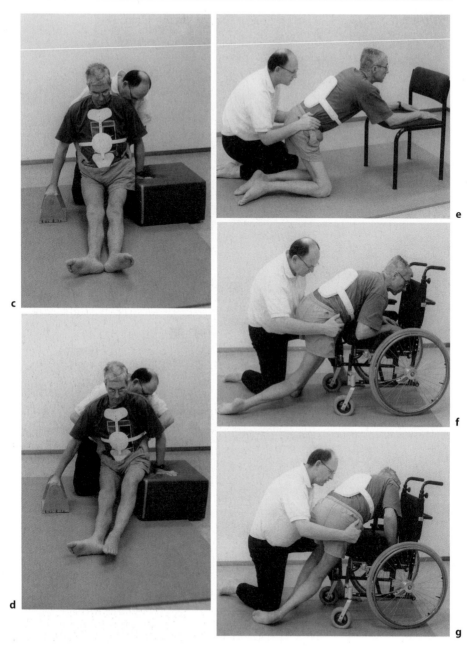

Fig. 11.38. Patient II. Incomplete paraplegia in the post-acute phase. **c, d** Long-sitting: push-ups and weight shift. **e–g** Transfer from floor into a chair and a wheelchair

Patient III   Ankylosing spondylitis (Spondylitis ankylopoetica)[1]
(Fig. 11.39)

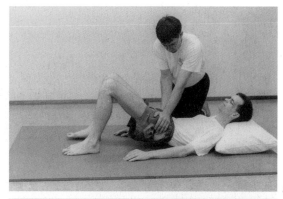

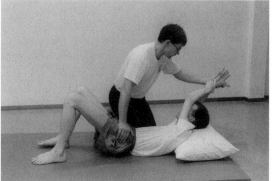

Fig. 11.39.a Bridging.
b Bridging combined with
lifting to the right.
c Kneeling with lifting

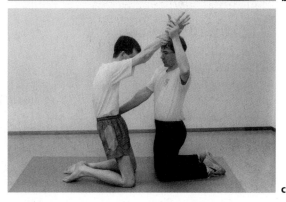

---

[1] Ankylosing spondylitis: The form of rheumatoid arthritis affecting the spine. It occurs predominantly in young males and produces pain and stiffness as a result of inflammation of the sacroiliac, intervertebral, and costovertebral joints. Aetiology is unknown. On-line Medical Dictionary (OMD), Academic Medical Publishing & Cancer WEB 1997–1998.

Patient IV   Incomplete tetraplegia with brachial plexus lesion (Fig. 11.40)

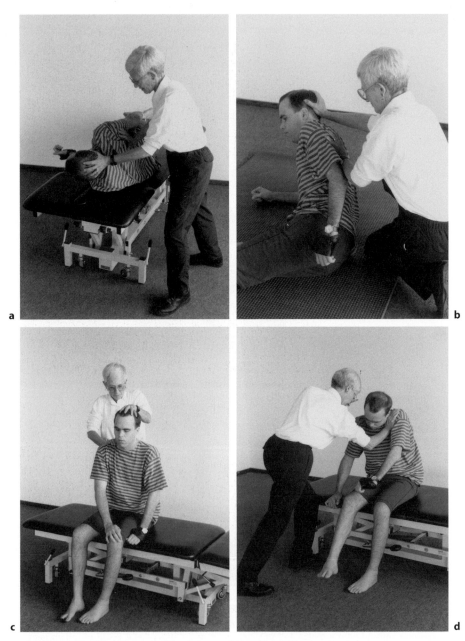

Fig. 11.40. a,b Side-lying and side-sitting. **c,d** Trunk stabilization in sitting

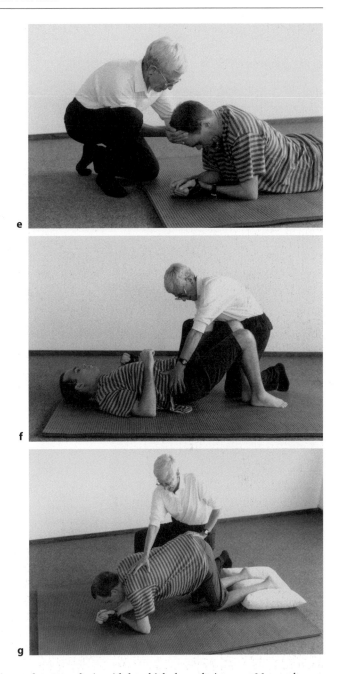

Fig. 11.40. Patient IV. Incomplete tetraplegia with brachial plexus lesion. **e–g** Mat work

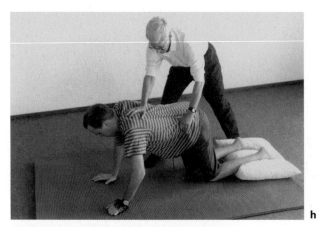

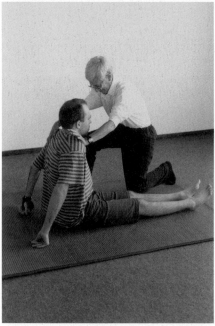

Fig. 11.40. Patient IV. Incomplete tetraplegia with brachial plexus lesion. **h, i** Mat work

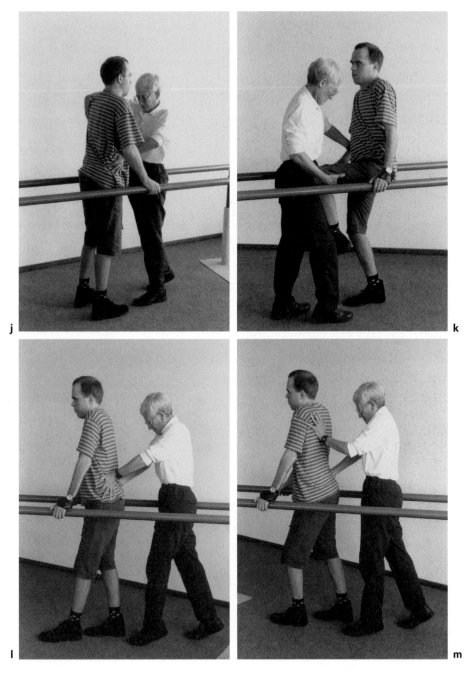

Fig. 11.40. Patient IV. Incomplete tetraplegia with brachial plexus lesion. **j–m** Standing and walking in parallel bars

Reference

VanSant AF (1991) Life-span motor development. In: Contemporary management of motor control problems. Proceedings of the II Step Conference. Foundation for Physical Therapy, Alexandria, VA

Further Reading

Portney LG, Sullivan PE, Schunk MC (1982) The EMG activity of trunk-lower extremity muscles in bilateral-unilateral bridging. Phys Ther 62:664
Schunk MC (1982) Electromyographic study of the peroneus longus muscle during bridging activities. Phys Ther 62:970–975
Sullivan PE, Portney LG, Rich CH, Langham TA (1982) The EMG activity of trunk and hip musculature during unresisted and resisted bridging. Phys Ther 62:662
Sullivan PE, Portney LG, Troy L, Markos PD (1982) The EMG activity of knee muscles during bridging with resistance applied at three joints. Phys Ther 62:648
Troy L, Markos PD, Sullivan PE, Portney LG (1982) The EMG activity of knee muscles during bilateral-unilateral bridging at three knee angles. Phys Ther 62:662

12 Gait Training

12.1 The Importance of Walking

Walking is a major goal for most patients. Effective walking requires the ability to change direction and to walk backward and sideways as well as forward. Being able to go up and down curbs, climb stairs and hills, and open and close doors increases the utility of the activity. To be totally functional the individual should be able to get down onto the ground and back up to standing again.

Walking must be so *automatic* that the person can turn his or her attention to the requirements of the environment, such as traffic, while continuing to walk. For walking to be safe the individual must be able to recover balance when disturbed, either by the act of walking or by outside forces. To walk more than a few steps requires gait that is as energy efficient as possible. To get around the house in a reasonable time requires less energy and speed than to walk around a supermarket or cross a street. The individual needs enough endurance and skill to walk the necessary distances at a practical speed (Lerner-Frankiel et al. 1986).

Knowing the elements of normal walking will help to analyze pathological gait and to plan therapeutic exercises.

12.2 Introduction: Basics of Normal Gait

12.2.1 The Gait Cycle (Figs. 12.1, 12.2)

To understand normal gait, we must know the basic terms associated with gait analysis. The gait cycle repeats a basic sequence of motions. This cycle of motions or gait cycle starts with heel strike of one leg and ends when the same foot strikes the ground again. It is divided in two major phases: the *stance* phase and the *swing* phase. The stance phase, the period the limb is on the ground, takes 60% of the cycle. The swing phase, the time when leg comes off the ground and moves in front of the body makes up the remaining 40% of the cycle.

The other divisions of the gait cycle are double limb support, when both feet are in contact with the floor, and single limb support, when only one foot contacts the floor. There are two periods of double support. The first occurs immediately after heel strike, the second prior to toe off. This second period of double limb support coincides with heel strike on the other side (Perry 1992).

The stance phase can be divided into initial contact (IC) also called heel strike (HS) when the heel contacts the floor first, loading response (LR), mid-stance (Mst), terminal stance (Tst) and pre-swing (Psw). Stance begins with the initial contact of the foot to the floor. Loading response begins immediately after foot contact. The body weight begins to shift onto this foot in preparation for the other leg to begin its swing phase. During this time the leg must not only accept the body weight but also maintain the forward motion of the body.

The next stance phases occur during the period of single limb support. Mid-stance begins when the other foot leaves the floor and continues through the time when the body weight is centered over the forefoot of the stance leg. Terminal stance begins when the heel begins to rise and continues until the other foot contacts the ground. During this time the body weight is in front of the supporting foot.

The final segment of the stance phase is pre-swing. The hip and knee are flexing, the ankle is plantar flexed and the toe is still in contact with the floor. The contralateral leg is now in contact with the ground and accepting the body weight.

The swing phases are initial swing (IS), mid-swing (MS) and terminal swing (TS) (Perry 1992). During initial swing the foot of the swinging limb is lifted clear of the floor by a combination of hip and knee flexion. The leg moves forward from the behind the body to a position opposite the supporting leg. During mid-swing the leg advances forward from its position opposite the stance limb. At the end of this phase the knee has started to extend, the tibia is vertical to the floor, and the ankle has dorsiflexed to a neutral position. In terminal swing the leg completes its forward motion by extension of the knee. The swing phase ends when the heel contacts the ground.

12.2.2 Trunk and Lower Extremity Joint Motion in Normal Gait

The center of gravity (CG) of the walking person is located in the pelvic area. During walking the CG moves both up and down, and right and left. The maximum upward excursion occurs at mid-stance and from there the CG drops to its lowest position during the phases of double support. The lateral displacement is towards the stance leg. Energy consumption during walking is partially controlled by the amount of CG movement. The most efficient motion is less than 10 cm (3 inches) of vertical and lateral motion.

Trunk and pelvic motions are also very important for an efficient gait pattern. During swing phase the ipsilateral pelvis rotates 4° forward and

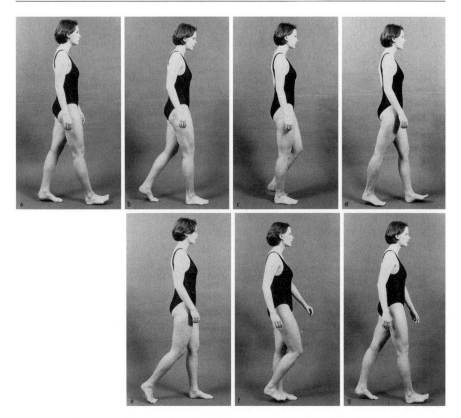

Fig. 12.1. The gait cycle (right leg, lateral view). **a** Heel strike right; **b** foot flat; **c** mid-stance; **d** heel off; **e** toe off right and pre-swing; **f** mid-swing; **g** heel strike after terminal swing

drops down just before the initial contact. By the end of stance the ipsilateral pelvis has rotated back by the same 4°. The rotation of the shoulder and the arm swing is opposite to the direction of rotation of the pelvis. Suppression of this counter rotation results in increased energy consumption and an inability to increase the velocity (Inman et al. 1981).

Stance (Figs. 12.1 a–e, 12.2 a–e)

At *heel strike* the ipsilateral pelvis is rotated forward, the hip is in 25–30° flexion. The knee is extended and the ankle is in neutral. For shock-absorption at heel strike, eccentric contraction of the ankle dorsiflexor muscles lower the forefoot to the floor and the knee moves into 15–20° flexion.

By *mid-stance* the hip, the knee and the ankle have moved into neutral (0°). As the body continues to progress forward the hip reaches a relative 20–30°

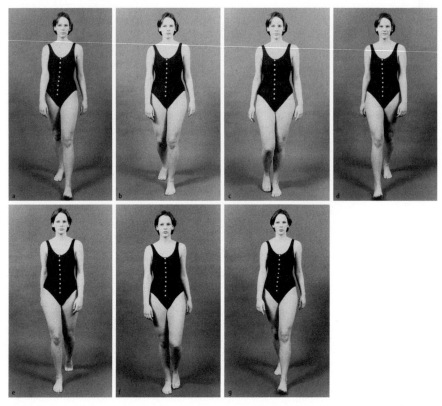

Fig. 12.2. The gait cycle (left leg, frontal view). **a** Heel strike left; **b** foot flat; **c** mid-stance; **d** heel off; **e** toe off left and pre-swing; **f** mid-swing; **g** heel strike after terminal swing

extension, due partially to the backward rotation of the pelvis. During the *terminal stance* and pre-swing, the hip and knee flex to prepare the swing. At the same time the ankle moves from 15° dorsal flexion at the start of heel-off to 20° plantar flexion at toe off.

Swing (Figs. 12.1 e–g,12.2 e–g)

Just before mid-swing the knee is in its maximum flexion of 65°, the hip is in 20° flexion and the ankle is in neutral. During the deceleration of the leg in terminal swing, the pelvis is rotated forward and is descending, the hip reaches 25° of flexion, the knee fully extends and the ankle remains in neutral.

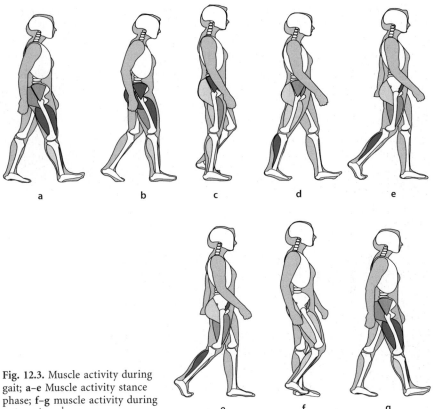

Fig. 12.3. Muscle activity during gait; **a–e** Muscle activity stance phase; **f–g** muscle activity during swing phase[1]

12.2.3 Muscle Activity During Normal Gait (Perry 1992)
(Fig. 12.3 a–g)

Muscle activity during forward walking works largely either to stabilize or decelerate the body segments. The momentum of the body as it moves forward provides most of the work for motion.

The *trunk flexor* and *extensor* muscles work throughout the gait cycle both to stabilize the trunk and to give the hip muscles a secure base for their work. The abdominals and the back extensor muscles stabilize the trunk in all planes. The trunk extensor muscles are more active after heel strike to stabilize the trunk during weight acceptance. The erector spinae are also active during the push off. The abdominals help to introduce the swing phase.

---

[1] Drawing by Ben Eisermann, Hoensbroek, muscle activity based on Perry J. 1992.

The *hip extensor* muscles are most active from the end of the swing phase, to decelerate the moving limb. Their activity continues through the initial contact and loading response as shock absorbers. There is essentially no activity of these muscles during mid-stance as the momentum of the body over the fixed foot provides the extension of the hip. The gluteus maximus is most active during heel strike and acts as a shock absorber by controlling the hip and knee extension and external rotation. During terminal stance these hip extensor muscles become active again to assist the propulsion.

The *hip abductor* muscles are active to stabilize the pelvis in the frontal plane (prevent excessive pelvic drop on the swing side). The abductor group is primarily active during heel strike and the early stance phase. The tensor faciae latae contracts more during the second part of stance.

The *quadriceps* and hamstring muscles also do most of their work at the end of swing through the beginning of stance. The *hamstrings* contract to assist in knee flexion at the end of the stance phase and to decelerate the lower leg (shank) at the end of the swing phase. They also assist the gluteus maximus in hip extension. The quadriceps are active at the end of swing and through the period of loading response as shock absorbers and to counteract the flexion torque during the loading response. Neither the hamstrings nor the quadriceps are active during mid-stance. Knee control during this time is managed by the calf group. The rectus femoris becomes active at the end of the stance phase together with the iliopsoas to introduce the forward swing of the leg.

The *pre-tibial muscle group* (dorsi-flexors) works during swing to raise the foot to neutral (0°) and then switch to eccentric work to lower the forefoot to the floor after heel strike. The *plantar flexor muscles* begin to work as soon as the foot is flat. First the soleus acts to control the tibia's forward motion. The tibial control provides passive knee extension and assists in hip extension. As the body continues its motion forward over the fixed foot the gastrocnemius contracts along with the soleus. At the end of stance all the plantar flexor muscles work to stabilize the ankle and allow the heel to rise up. This ankle restraint also aids the hip and knee flexion motion. During push off they act to propel the body forward.

12.3 Gait Analysis: Observation and Manual Evaluation

Adequate *joint range* of motion in the hip, knee, and ankle is needed for standing and walking to be practical. Limitation of motion at these joints, imposed by joint restrictions or by orthoses, will interfere with the normal swing and stance and decrease walking efficiency (Murray et al. 1964).

The individual needs *strength* in the muscles of the ankle, knee, hip, and trunk to stand up and walk without external support. Correct timing of the contraction and relaxation in these muscle groups is required for practical balance and gait (Horak and Nashner 1986; Eberhart et al. 1954). Exercises on the mats and treatment table are used to help bring the muscles to the level of strength needed for function.

To analyze the gait pattern start with an inspection in all three planes. In stance look for the alignment of the head and neck, shoulders and upper trunk, lumbar spine and pelvis, hips, knees and feet (Fig. 12.4). Inspection of the gait concentrates not only on the motion of the lower extremities but also on the symmetry of the leg and pelvic motion, the rotation of the upper trunk, and the arm swing. Check walking aids such as walkers, canes, orthoses or prostheses, and observe abnormal wear and tear on the shoes. Also note the velocity and endurance and whether the patient can walk independently.

Watch the patient's gait from the front and the back and from both sides. If possible have the patient walk backward and sideways as well as forward.

In the *sagittal* plane look for (Fig. 12.4 c):
- Excessive or decreased flexion and extension in the trunk, the hip, the knee and the ankle.
- Whether the right and left leg steps are of equal length and time duration.

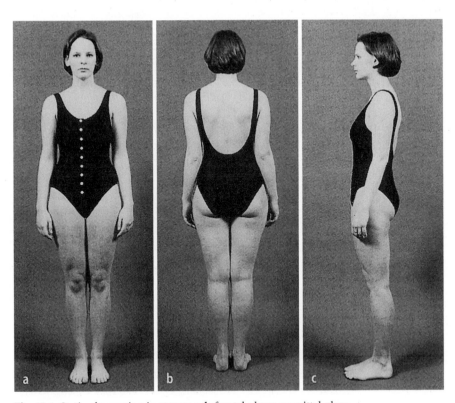

Fig. 12.4. Static observation in stance: **a, b** frontal plane; **c** sagittal plane

In the *frontal* plane look for asymmetry between the left and right sides (Fig. 12.4 a, b):

- Lateral trunk movement, pelvic tilting and dropping
- Reciprocal upper and lower trunk rotation and the arm swing
- The width of the gait base
- Abduction, adduction or circumduction of the hip
- Medio-lateral stability of the knee and ankle

For a *manual evaluation* of gait, place your hands on the person's pelvis and feel what is happening during unimpeded walking. Your hands go on the iliac crest as though you were resisting pelvic elevation. When evaluating, do not resist or approximate, just feel or assist if necessary (Fig. 12.5).

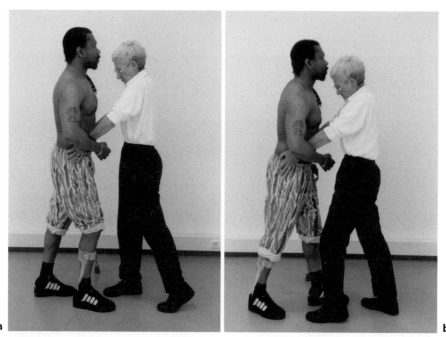

a   b

Fig. 12.5 a, b. Manual evaluation of gait without resistance or approximation; patient with right hemiplegia

12.4 The Theory of Gait Training

We use all the basic procedures and many of the techniques when working with our patients in standing and walking. Resistance, appropriately used, increases the patient's ability to balance and move. When the strong motions are resisted in standing and walking, irradiation will facilitate contraction of weaker trunk and lower extremity muscles. These weaker muscles will contract whether or not braces or other supports are used. There are occasions, however, when the patient's medical or physical condition does not allow successful work against resistance. In those instances the therapist gives whatever assistance is necessary but continues to use all the appropriate basic procedures such as voice, manual contact and even approximation if it is effective.

As the patient's ability increases he or she must be allowed and encouraged to stand and walk as independently as possible. During these practice sessions, no verbal or physical cueing should be given, and only the assistance necessary for safety. Allow patients to solve problems and correct mistakes on their own. Alternate resisted gait training with independent walking during a treatment session. After an activity is mastered, resisted work is used for strengthening.

Resisted gait activities can be used to treat specific joint and muscle dysfunctions in the upper and lower extremities. For example, exercise the lateral and medial ankle muscles by resisting sideways stepping. The shoulder, elbow, wrist, and hand are exercised when the patient holds the parallel bar while balancing or moving against resistance.

The PNF *techniques* are useful when working with the patient in gait. Rhythmic Initiation, Replication, and Combination of Isotonics help the patient to learn a new motion or to move to a position. Use of Stabilizing Reversals and Rhythmic Stabilization to facilitates stability. Using Dynamic Reversals will reduce fatigue and promote coordination. Use Relaxation techniques to improve functional mobility.

12.5 The Procedures of Gait Training

The primary emphasis in gait training is on the patient's trunk. Approximation through the pelvis during stance and stretch reflex to the pelvis during swing facilitate the muscles of the lower extremities and the trunk (S.S. Adler, unpublished, 1976). Proper placement of the hands allows the therapist to control the position of the patient's pelvis, moving it toward an anterior or posterior tilt as needed. When pelvic motion and stability are facilitated the legs can function more efficiently. Our hands can also be on the shoulder and on the head for stabilizing or facilitating trunk rotation.

Resistance to balance and motion is most effective when given in a diagonal direction. The therapist controls the direction of resistance by standing in the chosen diagonal. The therapist's body position also allows the use of body weight for approximation and resistance.

Resisted gait activities are *exaggerations* of normal motions. Large-amplitude body motions are resisted during weight shifting. During walking the pelvic motions are larger and the steps are higher. Resistance to the large motions helps the patient gain the strength and skill needed to stand and walk functionally.

12.5.1 Approximation and Stretch

Approximation facilitates contraction of the *extensor muscles* of the legs and promotes trunk stability. Correct timing of approximation during the stance phase is important. The first approximation comes at or just after heel strike to promote weight acceptance. The approximation may be repeated at any time during stance to maintain proper weight-bearing.

To approximate, place the heel (carpal ridge) of each hand on the anterior crest of the ilium, above the anterior superior iliac spine (ASIS). Your fingers point down and back in the direction of the force. Keep the patient's pelvis in a slight posterior tilt. The direction of the approximation force should go through the ischial tuberosities towards the patient's heels. Apply the approximation sharply and maintain it while adding resistance.

Precautions for the approximation
- Your wrists should be extended only a few degrees past neutral to avoid wrist injury.
- To avoid fatigue and shoulder pain, use your body weight to give the approximation force. Keep your elbows in a near-extended position so the body weight can come down through your arms (Fig. 12.6a).
- Your hands should stay on the crest of the ilium to prevent pain and bruising of the tissues of the abdomen and ASIS.

The *stretch reflex* facilitates contraction of the abdominal muscles and the flexor muscles of the swing leg. Correct timing of the stretch is when all the weight is off the foot (toe off).

To apply the stretch reflex at the pelvis, use the same grip as used for approximation. When the patient's foot is unweighted, stretch the pelvis down and back. The direction of the stretch is the same as for the pattern of anterior elevation of the pelvis.

Precautions for the stretch:
- Your hands should stay on the crest of the ilium and not slip down to the ASIS.
- The stretch should move the pelvis down and back. Do not rotate the patient's body around the stance foot.

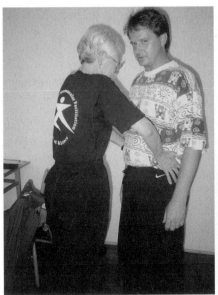
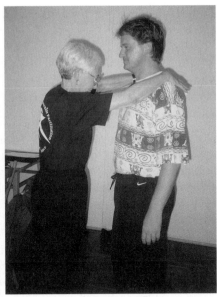

a   b

Fig. 12.6. a Approximation at the pelvis; **b** approximation at the scapula

12.5.2 Using Approximation and Stretch Reflex

Standing

Use approximation to facilitate balance and weight-bearing. Give resistance immediately to the resulting muscle contractions. The direction of the resistance determines which muscles are emphasized:

- Resistance directed diagonally backward facilitates and strengthens the anterior trunk and limb muscles.
- Resistance directed diagonally forward facilitates and strengthens the posterior trunk and limb muscles.
- Rotational resistance facilitates and strengthens all the trunk and limb muscles with an emphasis on their rotational component.

Approximation with resistance through the shoulder girdle places more demand on the upper trunk muscles. Put your hands on the top of the shoulder girdle to give the approximation. Be sure that the patient's spine is properly aligned before giving any downward pressure (Fig. 12.6b).

Walking

The walking descriptions below apply to walking forward with the therapist in front of the patient. The same principles hold true when the patient walks backward or sideways. When the patient walks backward, stand behind the patient and direct your pressure down and forward. For sideways balancing and walking stand to the side of the patient and direct your pressure down and laterally.

Swing Leg

Stretch and resistance to the upward and forward motion of the pelvis promotes both the pelvic motion and the hip flexion needed for swing. You can further facilitate hip flexion with timing for emphasis. Do this by blocking the pelvic motion until the hip begins to flex and the leg to swing forward. In normal gait the pelvic tilt during the first part of swing is minimal, but there has to be enough muscle tone in the trunk and abdominals to control a normal leg swing.

Stance Leg

Approximation combined with resistance to the forward motion of the pelvis facilitates and strengthens the extensor musculature. Give approximation in a downward and backward direction to the stance leg at or just after heel strike to promote weight acceptance. Approximate again at any time during the stance phase to maintain proper weight bearing.

12.6 Practical Gait Training

12.6.1 Preparatory Phase

A necessary part of a patient's gait training is learning to manage a wheelchair. These activities are a part of both gait and daily living training. Use all the basic procedures to help the patient gain skill in these activities. Repetition combined with resistance enables the patient to master the activities in the shortest possible time.

Managing the Wheelchair

The general activities are:
- Wheeling the chair
  - ▶ Forward (Fig. 12.7 a, b) and backward (Fig. 12.7 c, d) with resistance to the arms
  - ▶ Forward with resistance to the leg (Fig. 12.7 e, f)
- Locking and unlocking the brakes (Fig. 12.8)
- Removing and replacing the arm rests (Fig. 12.9 a, b)
- Managing the foot pedals (Fig. 12.10)

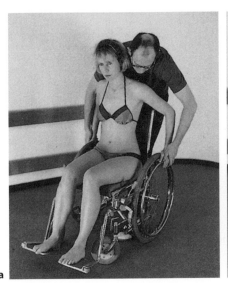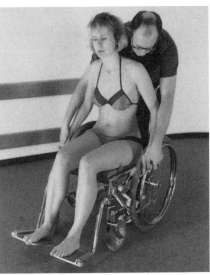

a   b

Fig. 12.7. Managing the wheelchair; a, b wheeling forward

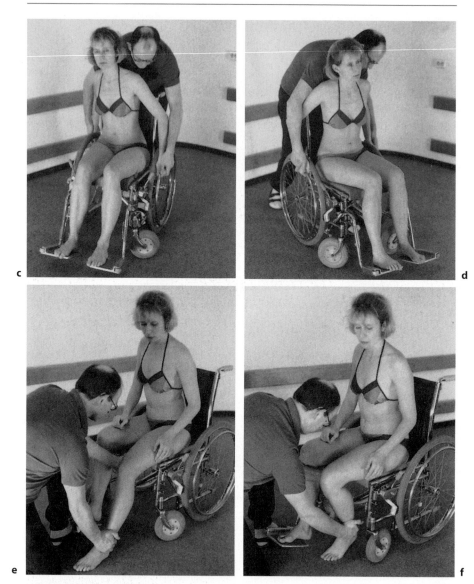

Fig. 12.7. Managing the wheelchair; **c,d** wheeling backward; **e,f** wheeling forward with resistance on the leg

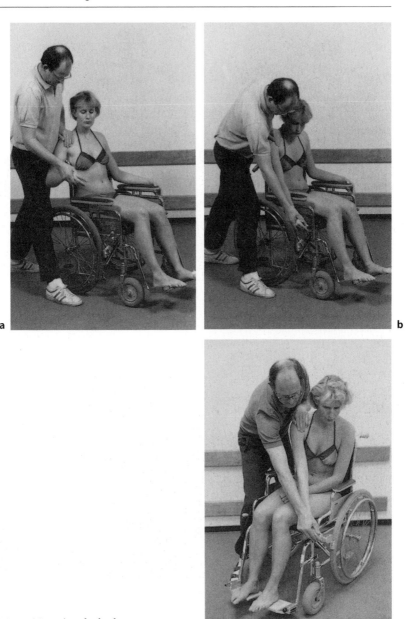

Fig. 12.8 a–c. Managing the brakes

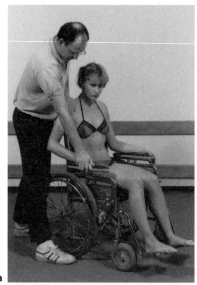
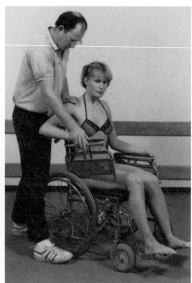

Fig. 12.9 a, b. Managing the armrests

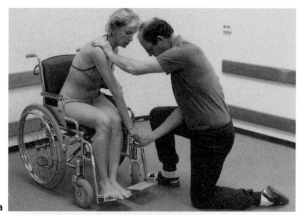

a

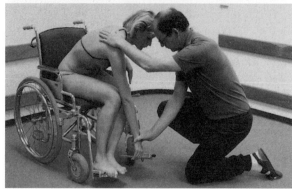

b

Fig. 12.10 a, b. Managing
the pedals

Sitting

It is necessary for the patient to be able to sit *upright* and move in a chair. Stretch and resistance at the pelvis can guide the patient into the proper erect posture with ischial weight bearing. Approximation and resistance at the scapula and head teaches and strengthens trunk stability. Use stretch reflex and resistance to the appropriate pelvic motions to teach the patient to move forward and backward in the chair. While working on these activities, evaluate the patient's strength and mobility. Treat any problems that limit function and reevaluate in a sitting position after treatment.

Example: You cannot get the patient's pelvis positioned for proper ischial weight bearing. Your evaluation shows that there is a limitation in the range of pelvic motion.

- Put the patient on mats and assess pelvic mobility using pelvic patterns.
- Treat the limitations in range and strength with exercises of pelvic and scapular patterns or a combination of the exercises with joint and soft tissue mobilization.
- After treatment, put the patient back into the wheelchair and reevaluate the pelvic position in sitting.

Sitting Activities

Getting into the Upright Sitting Position

- Use Combination of Isotonics with resistance at the head and shoulders to get the upper trunk into an erect position (Fig. 12.11).
- Use Rhythmic Initiation and stretch at the pelvis to achieve an anterior tilt.

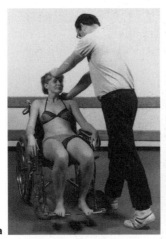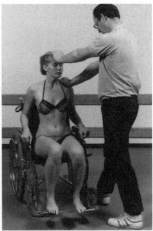

Fig. 12.11 a, b. Getting into an upright sitting position

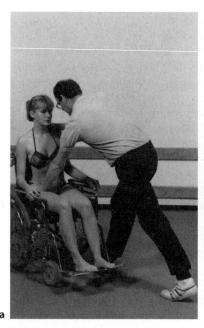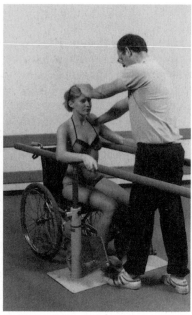

a   b

Fig. 12.12. Stabilizing the sitting position: **a** resistance at the pelvis and scapula; **b** resistance at head and scapula

Stabilizing in the Upright Position

Use Stabilizing Reversals (Fig. 12.12 a, b)
- At the head
- At the shoulders
- At the pelvis
- A combination of all of these

Moving in the Chair

Use Repeated Stretch, Rhythmic Initiation, and Isotonic Reversals (Slow Reversals)
- Pelvic anterior elevation for moving forward (Fig. 12.13)
- Pelvic posterior elevation for moving backward (Fig. 12.14, chair arm removed to show pelvic movement)

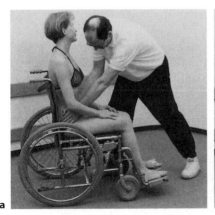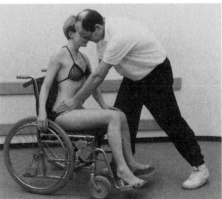

a   b

Fig. 12.13 a, b. Moving forward in the chair

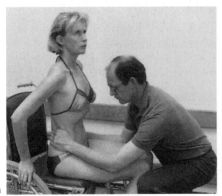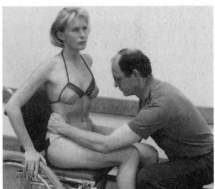

a   b

Fig. 12.14 a, b. Moving backward in the chair

12.6.2 Standing Up and Sitting Down

The following sections are an artificial grouping of activities. A treatment usually proceeds smoothly through all activities in a functional progression. The patient moves forward in the chair, stands up, gets his or her balance, and walks. You break down the activities as needed and work on those which are not yet functional or smooth.

Standing up is both a functional activity and a first stage in walking. The person should be able to stand up and sit down on surfaces of different heights. Although everyone varies in the way he or she gets from sitting to standing, the general motions can be summarized as follows (Nuzik et al. 1986):

- The first part of the activity (Fig. 12.15 a–c):
  - ▶ The head, neck, and trunk move into flexion.
  - ▶ The pelvis moves into a relative anterior tilt.
  - ▶ The knees begin to extend and move forward over the base of support.
- The last part (Fig. 12.15 d)
  - ▶ The head, neck, and trunk extend back toward a vertical position.
  - ▶ The pelvis goes from an anterior to a posterior tilt.
  - ▶ The knees continue extending and move backward as the trunk comes over the base of support.

Until studies bring other information, we assume that sitting down involves the reverse of these motions. Control comes from eccentric contraction of the muscles used for standing up.

To increase the patient's ability to stand up, place your hands on the patient's iliac crests (Fig. 12.16 a), rock or stretch the pelvis into a posterior tilt, and resist or assist as it moves into an anterior tilt. Rhythmic Initiation works well with this activity. Three repetitions of the motion are usually enough. On the third repetition give the command to stand up. Guide the pelvis up and into an anterior tilt as the patient moves toward standing. Assist the motion if that is needed, but resist when the patient can accomplish the act without help. As soon as the patient is upright guide the pelvis into the proper amount of posterior tilt. Approximate through the pelvis to promote weight bearing.

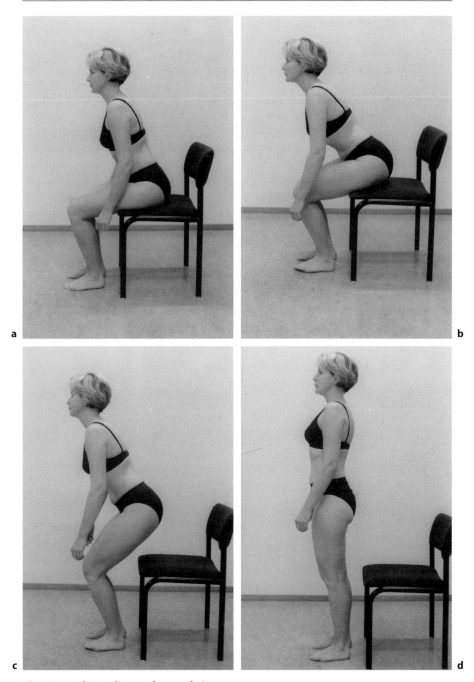

Fig. 12.15 a–d. Standing up from a chair

Getting to Standing

- Moving forward in chair: The same as practice in sitting.
- Placing hands: Use Rhythmic Initiation to teach patients where to put their hands. Use stabilizing contractions and Combination of Isotonics to teach them how to assist with their arms.
  - ▶ Using the parallel bars
  - ▶ Using the chair arms
- Rocking the pelvis: use Rhythmic Initiation and stretch to get the pelvis tilted forward (Fig. 12.16a).
- Coming to standing: guide and resist at the pelvis (Figs. 12.16, 12.17). Guide and resist at the shoulders if the patient cannot keep the upper trunk in proper alignment.

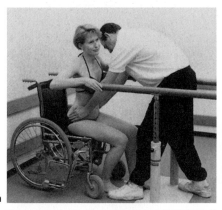

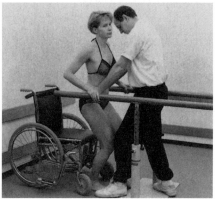

a   b

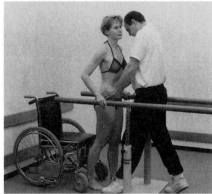

c

Fig. 12.16a–c. Getting to standing in parallel bars

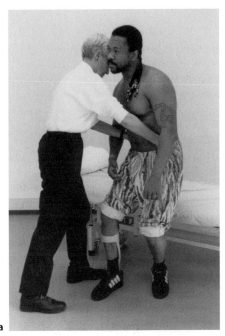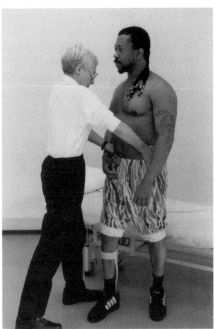

a   b

Fig. 12.17a, b. Standing up: patient with right hemiplegia

Sitting Down

- Placing hands to assist: Use the same techniques as in standing up to teach patients where to put their hands.
- Sitting down: Use resistance at the pelvis or pelvis and shoulders for eccentric control. When the patient is able, use Combination of Isotonics by having the patient stop part way down and then stand again.

12.6.3 Standing

Stand in a diagonal in front of the leg that is to take the patient's weight initially. Guide the patient to that side and use approximation and stabilizing resistance at the pelvis to promote weight-bearing on that leg (Fig. 12.17b; Fig. 12.16c). If weight is to be borne equally on both legs stand directly in front of the patient.

Weight Acceptance

- Combine approximation through the pelvis on the strong side with stabilizing resistance at the pelvis.
- Combine approximation through the pelvis on the weaker side (knee blocked if necessary) with stabilizing resistance at the pelvis.

Stabilization

- Combine Approximation and Stabilizing Reversals at the pelvis for the lower trunk and legs (Fig. 12.18 a).
- Combine Approximation and Stabilizing Reversals at the shoulders for the upper and lower trunk (Fig. 12.18 b).
- Using Combination of Isotonics with small motions or Stabilizing Reversals, resist balance in all directions. Work at the head, the shoulders, the pelvis, and combination of these.

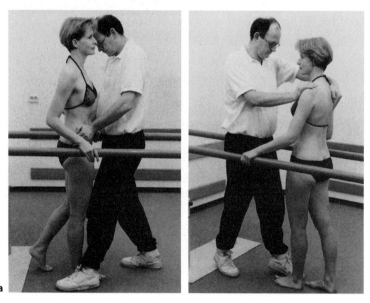

Fig. 12.18 a, b. Stabilization at the pelvis and on the shoulders

One-Leg Standing

Use this activity to promote weight bearing in stance and to facilitate pelvic and hip motion in swing. The patient stands on one leg with the other hip flexed. The flexed hip should be above 90° if possible, to facilitate hip extension on the other leg. If the patient is not able to hold up the flexed leg, assist by placing the patient's knee above your pelvis and giving a compressive force to hold the leg in place (Fig. 12.19b). Alternate the weight-bearing leg frequently to avoid fatigue.

Emphasis on Stance Leg

- Approximate through the pelvis to encourage weight bearing (Fig. 12.19a).
- Use Combination of Isotonics with small motions or Stabilizing Reversals at the pelvis to resist balance in all directions.

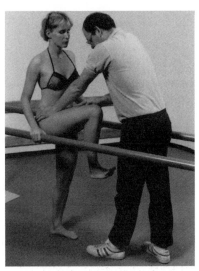

Fig. 12.19. Standing on one leg; a emphasis on stance leg

a

Emphasis on Swing Leg

- Use Repeated Stretch with resistance to facilitate anterior elevation of the pelvis on that side (Fig. 12.19 b, c).
- Use Combination of Isotonics to facilitate hip flexion.

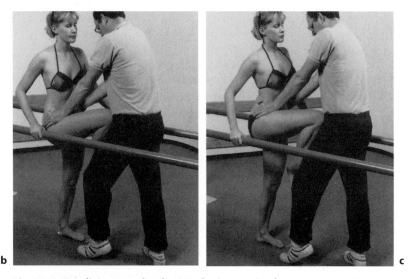

b   c

Fig. 12.19. Standing on one leg; **b, c** emphasis on swing leg

Weight Shifting

Use this activity both as a preliminary to stepping and to exercise specific motions in the lower extremity. Exaggerated weight shift forward or laterally exercises the hip hyperextension and lateral motions, knee stability, and ankle motion.

Start the weight shift activity by stabilizing the patient on one leg. Then resist as he or she shifts weight to the other leg. Using approximation and resistance, stabilize the patient in the new position. You can complete this exercise in one of two ways:

- By resisting eccentric contraction as the patient allows you to push him or her slowly back over the other leg.
- By resisting concentric contractions while the patient actively shifts weight to the other leg. In this case, you must move your hands to give resistance to the motion.

Weight Shift from Side to Side

- Stabilizing resistance with weight on both legs
- Resistance to sideways weight shift
- Approximation and resistance on weight-bearing side
- Resisted eccentric or concentric return:
  - ▶ Eccentric: keep your hands positioned to resist the original weight shift.
  - ▶ Concentric: move your hands to the opposite side of the pelvis; resist an antagonistic weight shift.

Weight Shift Forward and Backward (Stride Position)
(Fig 12.20)

When working on this activity it is important for the patient to shift the whole pelvis and trunk forward and backward. Do not allow the patient to come forward in a sideways position. Stand in front of the patient to emphasize forward weight shift, and behind to emphasize backward weight shift. As always, stand in the line of the patient's motion. The example below is for shifting forward; reverse the directions for shifting backward.

Example

The patient is standing with weight on the left leg and the right leg forward. You stand in a diagonal stride position in front of the patient's right leg. Your right foot is forward in front of the patient's back foot. Your weight is on your forward foot.

- Stabilize: use approximation and resistance to stabilize the patient on the back leg (Fig. 12.20 a)

- Resist: give diagonal resistance as the patient's weight shifts from the back to the front leg. Let the patient's movement push you back over your rear leg (Fig. 12.20 b).
- Stabilize: give approximation through the left (front) leg combined with bilateral resistance to stabilize the patient on the front leg. Use your body weight to give the resistance.
- Resist: give diagonal resistance to eccentric or concentric work to return the patient's weight to his back leg:
  ▶ Eccentric: keep your hands positioned on the anterior superior iliac crests.
  ▶ Concentric: move your hands to the posterior superior iliac crests.

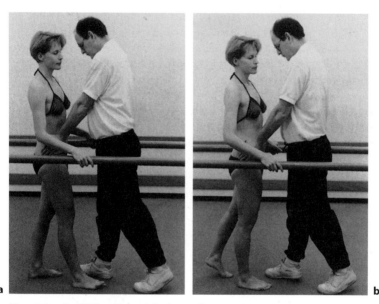

a   b

Fig. 12.20 a, b. Shifting the weight forward

Repeated Stepping (Forward and Backward)
(Fig. 12.20 c, d)

This activity goes with weight shifting. You may have the patient shift weight three or four times before stepping or ask for a step following each weight shift. As the patient steps, you shift your body to place it in the line of the new stance leg. Use this activity to exercise any part of swing or stance that needs work. You may modify the activity to do repeated stepping sideways.

Example
- Repeated stepping forward and back with the right leg.
  - ▶ Stabilize on the back (right) leg.
  - ▶ Resist the weight shift to the forward (left) leg.
  - ▶ Stabilize on the forward leg.
  - ▶ Stretch and resist: when the patient's weight is on the left leg, stretch the right side of the pelvis down and back. Resist the upward and forward motion of the pelvis to facilitate the forward step of the right leg. As the patient steps with the right leg, you step back with your left leg.
  - ▶ Stabilize on the forward leg.
- Resist the weight shift back to the left leg:
  - ▶ Eccentric: maintain the same grip as you push the patient slowly back over the left leg.
  - ▶ Concentric: shift your grip to the posterior pelvic crest and resist the patient shifting his or her weight back over the left leg.
- Resist a backward step with the right leg:
  - ▶ Eccentric: tell the patient to step back slowly while you maintain the same grip and try to push the pelvis and leg back rapidly.
  - ▶ Concentric: shift your grip to the posterior pelvic crest, then stretch and resist an upward and backward pelvic motion to facilitate a backward step with the right leg.

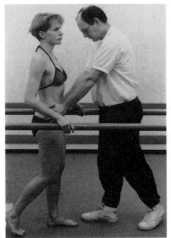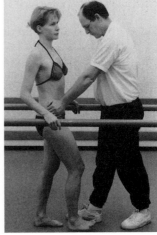

c   d

Fig. 12.20 c, d. Stepping forward

12.6.4 Walking

After weight shifting and repeated stepping, it is time to put all the parts
together and let the patient walk. When the objective of the walk is
evaluation or function, give the patient just enough support to maintain
safety. When the objective is to strengthen and reeducate, use approximation,
stretch, and resistance as you did with weight shift and repeated stepping.

> **!** Caution: resisted walking interrupts the patient's momentum
> and coordination and decreases velocity.

Forward

Standing in Front of the Patient

Mirror the patient's steps. As the patient steps forward with the right leg you
step back with your left. Use the same procedures and techniques as you
used for repeated stepping (Fig. 12.21 a, b).

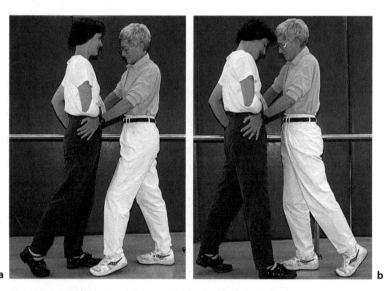

a   b

Fig. 12.21. Forward gait. **a, b** Therapist in front of the patient

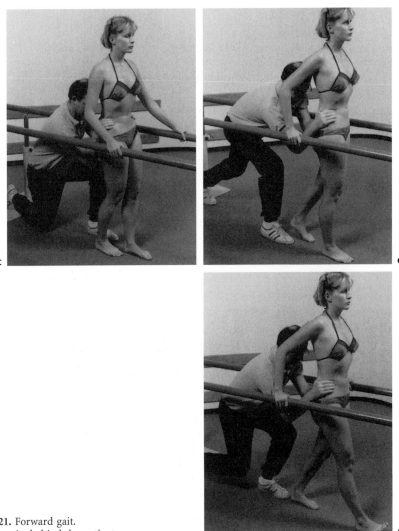

Fig. 12.21. Forward gait.
c–e Therapist behind the patient

Standing Behind the Patient (Fig. 12.21 c–e)

Both you and the patient step with the same leg. When standing behind, your fingers are on the iliac crest. Your hands and forearms form a line that points down through the ischial tuberosities towards the patient's heels. Your forearms press against the patients gluteal muscles (Fig. 12.21c).

Standing behind is advantageous when:
- The patient is much taller than you are: you can use your body weight to pull down and back on the pelvis for approximation, stretch, and resistance.
- You want to give the patient an unobstructed view forward.
- The patient is using a walker or other walking aid.

Backward (Fig. 12.22)

Walking backward is a necessary part of functional walking. It requires trunk control and exercises hip hyperextension in swing. Backward walking also serves to facilitate forward walking by acting as the technique Reversal of Antagonists.

- Stand behind the patient. Place the heel of your hand on the posterior superior iliac crest and give pressure down and forward.
- The patient must maintain an upright trunk while walking backward.

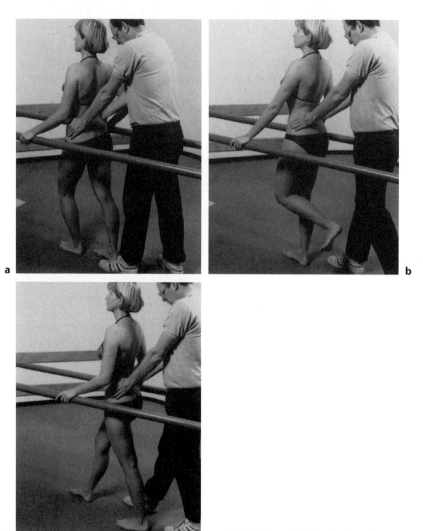

Fig. 12.22 a–c. Walking backward

Sideways
(Fig. 12.23, walking sideways; Fig. 12.24, braiding)

The ability to walk sideways is needed when maneuvering in narrow places. Walking sideways exercises the lateral muscles of the trunk and legs: Stand so the patient walks towards you. Give approximation, stretch, and resistance through the pelvis. If the upper trunk needs stabilizing, place one hand on the lateral aspect of the shoulder.

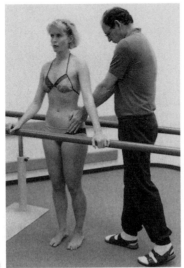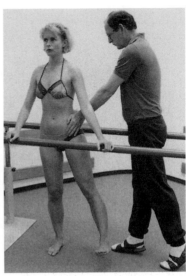

a   b

Fig. 12.23 a, b. Walking sideways

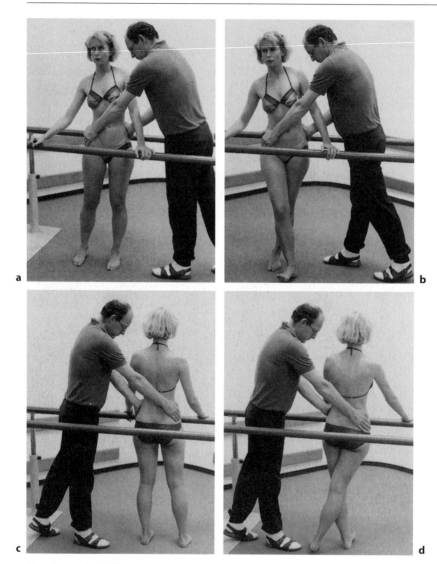

Fig. 12.24 a–d. Braiding

12.6.5 Other Activities

Here we illustrate some other activities we consider important for the patient to master. Use the procedures and techniques that are appropriate for each situation.

- Walking outside the bars (Fig. 12.25)
- Walking with crutches (Fig. 12.26)
- Going up and down stairs (Fig. 12.27)
- Going up and down curbs (Fig. 12.28) Curbs are one step without a railing.
- Going down and getting up from the floor. (We cover this activity in Chap. 11, but also consider it an important part of walking.)

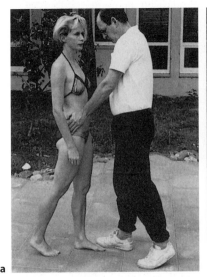 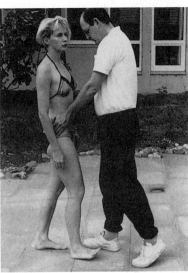

a   b

Fig. 12.25 a, b. Walking outside the parallel bars

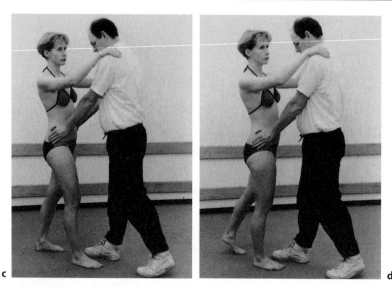

Fig. 12.25 c, d. Walking outside the parallel bars

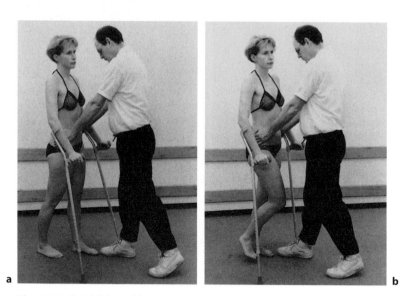

Fig. 12.26 a, b. Walking with crutches

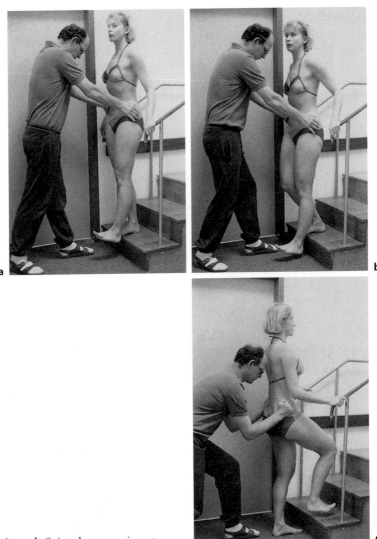

Fig. 12.27. Stairs. **a, b** Going down; **c** going up

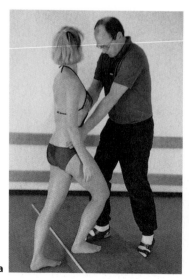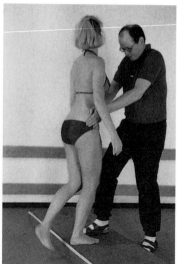

a   b

Fig. 12.28 a, b. Going up a curb

12.7 Patient Cases in Gait Training

Patient I. Patient with right hemiplegia (Fig. 12.29 a–f)

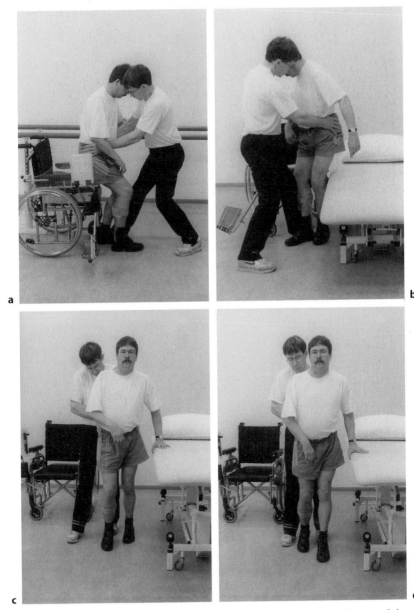

Fig. 12.29. a Getting to standing; **b** transfer from wheelchair to table; **c, d** facilitation of the stance phase on the hemiplegic leg

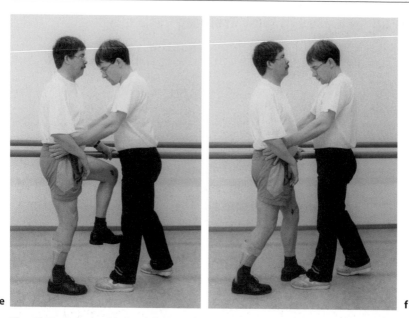

e   f

Fig. 12.29. Patient with hemiplegia. **e,f** stance on the involved leg with emphasis on hip extension and knee control

Patient II. Patient with ankylosing spondylitis (Fig. 12.30 a–c).

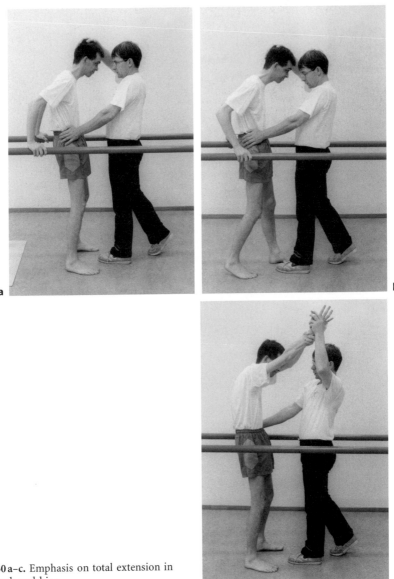

Fig. 12.30 a–c. Emphasis on total extension in neck, trunk and hips

Patient III. Patient with fracture of the right tibia, external fixation and partial weight acceptance (Fig. 12.31 a–c).

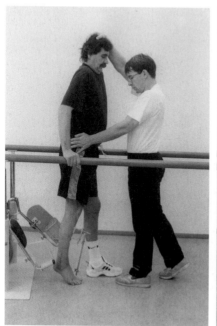

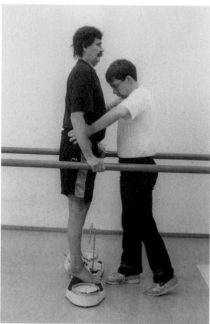

a

b

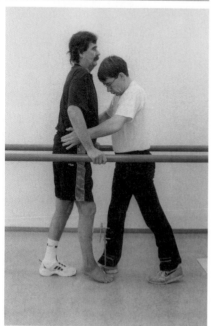

c

Fig. 12.31. a Emphasis on hip extension with partial weight support; **b** weight-bearing up to 50% or 40 kg (80 pounds) on the involved leg; **c** exercise of weight shift forward

Patient IV. Patient with below-knee amputation of the left leg (Fig. 12.32a–e).

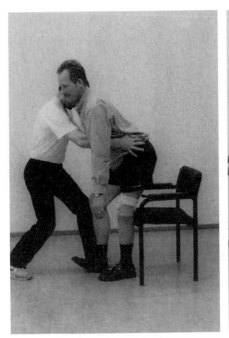

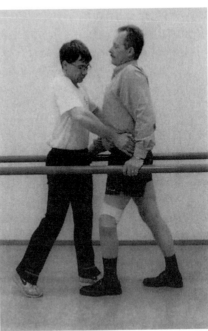

a

b

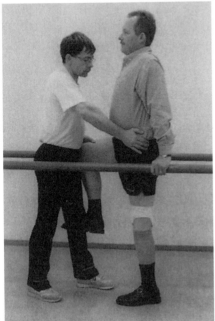

c

Fig. 12.32 a–c. a Standing up; **b** weight shift on the prosthesis with knee control; **c** standing on prosthetic leg, emphasis on hip and knee extension during stance phase

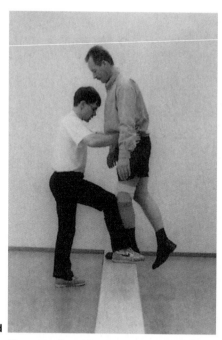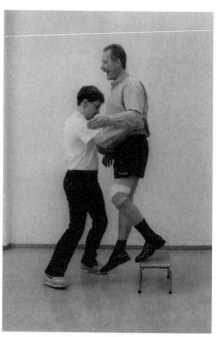

d   e

Fig. 12.32 d, e. d stepping up, control with prosthetic leg; **e** stepping down, control with prosthetic leg

References

Adler SS (1976) Influence of "Joint Approximation" on lower extremity extensor muscles: an EMG study. Unpublished thesis presented at APTA annual conference, New Orleans

Beckers D, Deckers J (1997) Ganganalyse und Gangschulung, Springer Verlag, Berlin Heidelberg New York

Eberhart HD, Inman VT, Bresler B (1954) The principal elements in human locomotion. In: Klopteg PE, Wilson PD (eds) Human limbs and their substitutes. McGraw-Hill, New York

Horak FB, Nashner LM (1986) Central programming of postural movements: adaptation to altered support-surface configurations. J Neurophysiol 55 (6):1369–1381

Inman VT, Ralston HJ, Todd F (1981) Human walking. Williams & Wilkins, Baltimore

Lerner-Frankiel MB, Vargas S, Brown M, Krusell L (1986) Functional community ambulation: what are your criteria? Clin Management 6 (2):12–15

Murray MP, Drought AB, Kory RC (1964) Walking patterns of normal men. J Bone Joint Surg [A]:335–360

Nuzik S, Lamb R, VanSant A, Hirt S (1986) Sit-to-stand movement pattern, a kinematic study. Phys Ther 66 (11):1708–1713

Perry J (1992) Gait analysis, normal and pathological function. Slack, NJ

Further Reading

Posture Control and Movement

Finley FR, Cody KA (1969) Locomotive characteristics of urban pedestrians. Arch Phys Med Rehabil 51:423–426

Gahery Y, Massion J (1981) Co-ordination between posture and movement. Trends Neurosci 4:199–202

Nashner LM (1980) Balance adjustments of humans perturbed while walking. J Neurophysiol 44:650–664

Nashner LM (1982) Adaptation of human movement to altered environments. Trends Neurosci 5:358–361

Nashner LM, Woollacott M (1979) The organization of rapid postural adjustments of standing humans: an experimental-conceptual model. In: Talbott RE, Humphrey DR (eds) Posture and movement. Raven, New York

Woollacott MH, Shumway-Cook A (1990) Changes in posture control across the life span – a systems approach. Phys Ther 70:799–807

Gait

Inman VT, Ralston HJ, Todd F (1981) Human walking. Williams and Wilkins, Baltimore

Kettelkamp DB, Johnson RJ, Schmidt GL, et al (1970) An electrogoniometric study of knee motion in normal gait. J Bone Joint Surg [A] 52:775–790

Lehmann JF (1990) Gait analysis, diagnosis and management. In: Krusens handbook of physical medicine and rehabilitation, Saunders, Philadelphia, pp 108–125

Lehmann JF (1990) Lower extremity orthotics. In: Krusens Handbook of physical medicine and rehabilitation. Saunders, Philadelphia, pp 602–646

Mann RA, Hagy JL, White V, Liddell D (1979) The initiation of gait. J Bone Joint Surg [A] 61:232–239

McFadyen BJ, Winter DA (1988) An integrated biomechanical analysis of normal stair ascent and descent. J Biomech 21:733–744

Murray MP, Kory RC, Sepic SB (1970) Walking patterns of normal women. Arch Phys Med Rehabil 51:637–650

Murray MP, Drought AB, Kory RC (1964) Walking patterns of normal men. J Bone Joint Surg [A] 46:335–360

Nashner LM (1976) Adapting reflexes controlling the human posture. Exp Brain Res 26:59–72

The Pathokinesiology Service and The Physical Therapy Department, Ranch Los Amigos Medical Center (1993) Observational Gait Analysis. Los Amigos Research and Education Institute Inc, Downey CA

Smidt G (1990) Gait in rehabilitation. Churchill Livingstone, New York

Sutherland DH (1966) An electromyographic study of the plantar flexors of the ankle in normal walking on the level. J Bone Joint Surg [A] 48:66–71

Sutherland DH, Cooper L, Daniel D (1980) The role of the ankle plantar flexors in normal walking. J Bone Joint Surg [A] 62:354–363

Sutherland DH, Olshen R, Cooper L, Woo SLY (1980) The development of mature gait. J Bone Joint Surg 62:336–353

Winter D (1989) The biomechanics and motor control of human gait. University of Waterloo Press, Waterloo

Wittle M (1991) Gait analysis: an introduction. Butterworth-Heinemann, Oxford

13 Vital Functions

13.1 Introduction

Therapy for the vital functions includes exercises for the face, tongue, breathing, and swallowing. Treatment of these areas is of particular importance when facial weakness, swallowing, and respiratory difficulties are involved. You can do breathing and facial exercises anytime. Breathing exercises are particularly useful for active recuperation when a patient becomes fatigued from other activities and for relaxation if the patient is tense or in pain.

13.1.1 Stimulation and Facilitation

Use the same procedures and techniques when treating problems in breathing, swallowing, and facial motion as when treating other parts of the body. Using the stretch reflex and resistance promote muscle activity and increase strength. Proper grip and pressure will guide and facilitate the movements. Additional facilitation can be achieved by using *ice* for facilitation (quick ice). Use two or three quick, short strokes with the ice on the skin overlying the muscles, on the tongue, or inside the mouth.

Use bilateral movements (both sides together) when exercising the face. Contraction of the muscles on the stronger or more mobile side will facilitate and reinforce the action of the more involved muscles. Timing for emphasis, by preventing full motion on the stronger side, will further promote activity in the weaker muscles.

13.2 Facial Muscles

The muscles of the face have many functions, including facial expression, jaw motion, protecting the eyes, aiding in speech (Fig. 13.1). The specific actions of the facial muscles are not detailed here as they are amply covered by books on muscle testing. Co-treatment with a speech therapist, if available, is recommended.

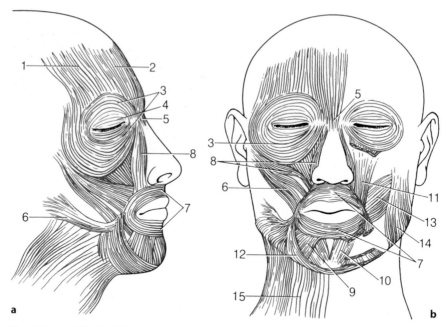

Fig. 13.1 a, b. The facial muscles [from: Feneis H (1967) Anatomisches Bildwörterbuch. Thieme, Stuttgart, modified by B. Eisermann]. Numbers correlate with muscles on the following pages

General principles for treating the face include:
- Gross motions are mass opening and mass closing.
- There are two general facial areas, the eyes and forehead, and the mouth and jaw. The nose works with both general areas.
- Facial motions are exercised in diagonal patterns.
- The face should be treated bilaterally; the stronger side reinforces motions on the weaker side.

Contraction of the muscles on the stronger or more mobile side will facilitate and reinforce the action of the more involved muscles. Timing for emphasis, by preventing full motion on the stronger side, will further promote activity in the weaker muscles.
- Strong motions in other parts of the body will reinforce the facial muscles. This occurs in our everyday lives. For example, when trying with effort to open a jar, you will unconsciously contract your facial muscles.
- Functionally, the facial muscles must work against gravity; this must be considered when choosing a position for treatment.
- A mirror can help patients control their facial movements (Fig. 13.2).

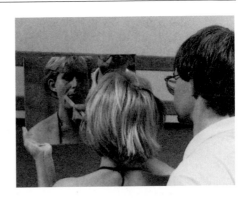

Fig. 13.2. A mirror can help patients control their facial movements

1. M. Epicranius (Frontalis) (Fig. 13.3)

Command. "Lift your eyebrows up, look surprised, wrinkle your forehead."

Apply resistance to the forehead, pushing caudally and medially.
This motion works with eye opening. It is reinforced with neck extension.

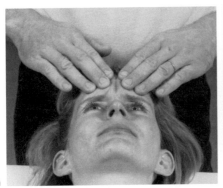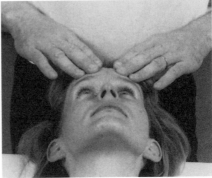

a   b

Fig. 13.3a,b. Facilitation of m. epicranius (frontalis)

2. M. Corrugator (Fig. 13.4)

Command. "Frown, pull your eyebrows down."

Give resistance just above the eyebrows diagonally in a cranial and lateral direction. This motion works with eye closing.

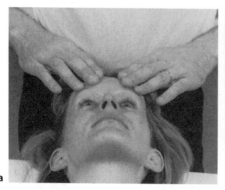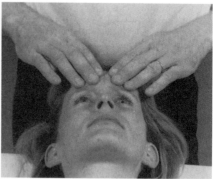

a   b

Fig. 13.4a,b. Facilitation of m. corrugator

3. M. Orbicularis Oculi (Fig. 13.5)

Command. "Close your eyes."

Use separate exercises for the upper and lower eyelids. Give gentle diagonal resistance to the eyelids. Avoid putting pressure on the eyeballs.

The previous two motions are facilitated by neck flexion.

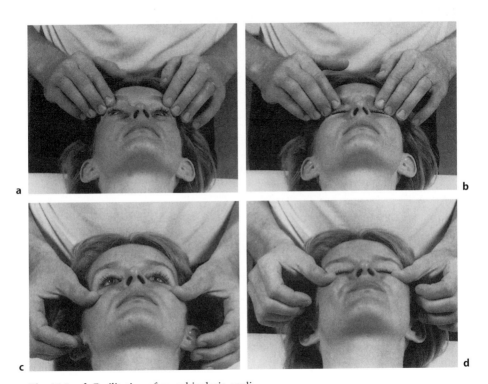

Fig. 13.5 a–d. Facilitation of m. orbicularis oculi

4. M. Levator Palpebrae Superioris (Fig. 13.6)

Command. "Open your eyes. Look up."

Give resistance to the upper eyelids. Resistance to eyebrow elevation will reinforce the action.

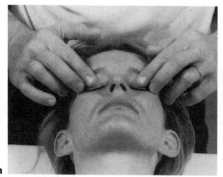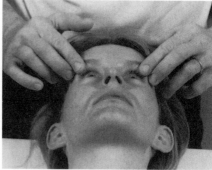

a   b

Fig. 13.6a,b. Facilitation of m. levator palpebrae superioris

5. M. Procerus (Fig. 13.7)

Command. "Wrinkle your nose."

Apply resistance next to the nose diagonally down and out.
This muscle works with m. corrugator and with eye closing.

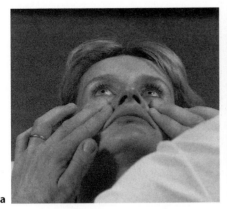 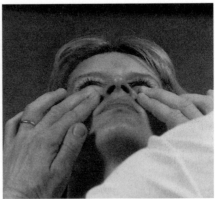

Fig. 13.7 a, b. Facilitation of m. procerus

6. *M. Risorius and M. Zygomaticus Major* (Fig. 13.8)

Command. "Smile."

Apply resistance to the corners of the mouth medially and slightly downward (caudally).

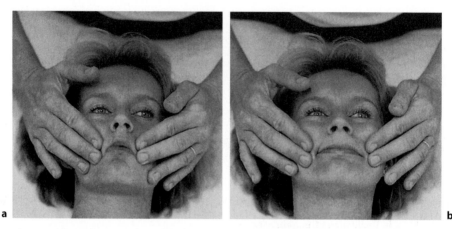

a   b

Fig. 13.8 a, b. Facilitation of m. risorius and m. zygomaticus major

7. *M. Orbicularis Oris* (Fig. 13.9)

Command. "Purse your lips, whistle, say 'prunes'."

Give resistance laterally and upward to the upper lip, laterally and downward to the lower lip.

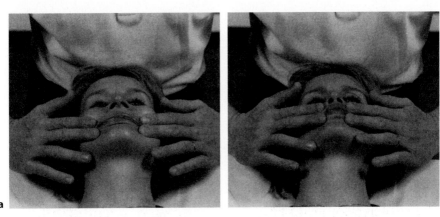

a   b

Fig. 13.9 a, b. Facilitation of m. orbicularis oris

8. M. Levator Labii Superioris (Fig. 13.10)

Command. "Lift your upper lip, show your upper teeth."

Apply resistance to the upper lip, downward and medially.

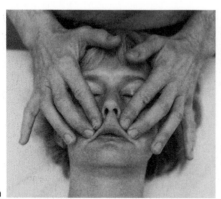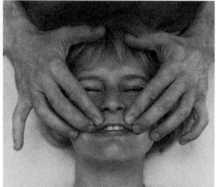

a   b

Fig. 13.10a,b. Facilitation of m. levator labii superioris

9. M. Depressor Labii Inferioris

Command. "Push your lower lip downwards, show your lower teeth."

Apply resistance upward and medially to the lower lip.
This muscle and the platysma work together.

10. M. Mentalis (Fig. 13.11)

Command. "Wrinkle your chin."

Apply resistance down and out at the chin.

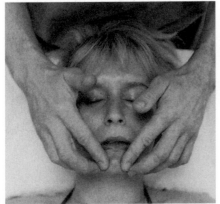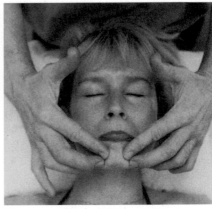

a   b

Fig. 13.11 a, b. Facilitation of m. mentalis

11. *M. Levator Anguli Oris* (Fig. 13.12)

Command. "Pull the corner of your mouth up, a small smile".

Push down and in at the corner of the mouth.

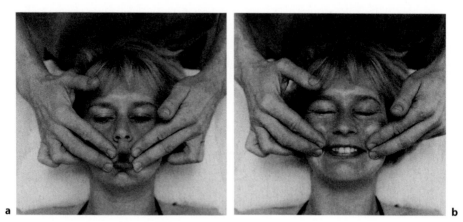

a　　　　　　　　　　　　　　　　　　　　　　　　　　　　**b**

Fig. 13.12a,b. Facilitation of m. levator anguli oris

12. *M. Depressor Anguli Oris* (Fig. 13.13)

Command. "Push the corners of your mouth down, look sad."

Give resistance upwards and medially to the corners of the mouth.

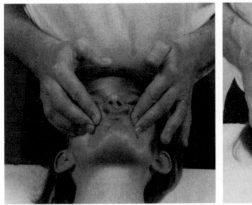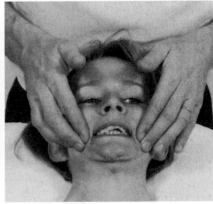

a   b

Fig. 13.13 a, b. Facilitation of m. depressor anguli oris

13. M. Buccinator (Fig. 13.14)

Command. "Suck your cheeks in, pull in against the tongue blade."

Apply resistance on the inner surface of the cheeks with your gloved fingers or a dampened tongue blade. The resistance can be given diagonally upward or diagonally downward as well as straight out.

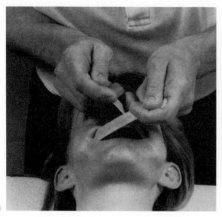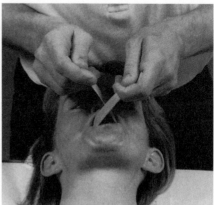

a   b

Fig. 13.14 a, b. Facilitation of m. buccinator

14. M. Masseter Temporalis (Fig. 13.15)

Command. "Close your mouth, bite."

Apply resistance to the lower jaw diagonally downward to the right and to the left. Resist in a straight direction if diagonal resistance disturbs the temporomandibular joint. Resistance to the neck extensor muscles reinforces active jaw closing.

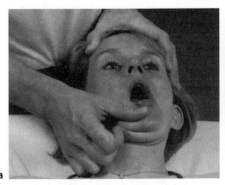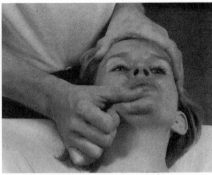

a b

Fig. 13.15 a, b. Facilitation of m. masseter and m. temporalis

15. M. Infrahyoid and M. Suprahyoid (Fig. 13.16)

Command. "Open your mouth."

Give resistance under the chin either diagonally or in a straight direction
(see Chapter 14). Resistance to the neck flexor muscles reinforces active jaw
opening.

> **Note: When exercising mouth opening and closing, the skull remains still,
> the mandible moves in relation to the skull.**

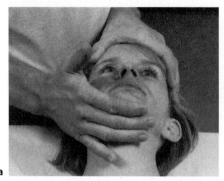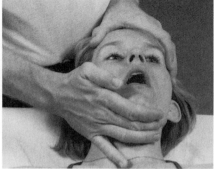

a   b

Fig. 13.16 a, b. Facilitation of m. infrahyoidei and mm. suprahyoid

16. M. Platysma (Fig. 13.17)

Command. "Pull your chin down."

Give resistance under the chin to prevent the mouth from opening.
Resistance may be diagonal or in a straight plane as in Fig. 13.17.
Resisted neck flexion reinforces this muscle.

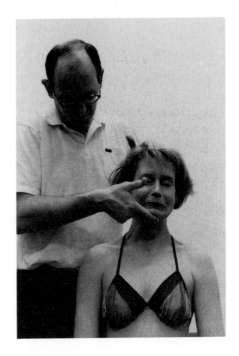

Fig. 13.17. Exercising the platysma

17. Intrinsic Eye Muscles

Eye motions are reinforced by resisted head and trunk motion in the desired
direction.

To reinforce eye motion down and to the right, resist neck flexion to the
right and ask the patient to look in that direction. To reinforce lateral eye
motion resist full rotation of the head to that side and tell the patient to look
to that side. Give the patient a definite target to look at with your command.

Example: "Tuck your head down (to the right) and look at your right knee."

13.3 Tongue Movements

Use a tongue blade or your gloved fingers to stimulate and resist tongue movements. Wet the tongue blade to make it less irritating to the tissues. Ice the tongue to increase the stimulation. Sucking on an ice cube permits patients to stimulate tongue and mouth function on their own.

We have illustrated the following tongue exercises:
- Sticking the tongue out straight (Fig. 13.18 a)
- Sticking the tongue out to the left and the right (Fig. 13.18 b)
- Touching the nose with the tongue (Fig. 13.18 c)
- Touching the chin with the tongue (Fig. 13.18 d)
- Rolling the tongue. (This motion is genetically controlled. Not all people can do it.) (Fig. 13.18 e)

Other tongue motions which should be exercised include:
- Humping the tongue (needed to push food back in the mouth in preparation for swallowing)
- Moving the tongue laterally inside the mouth
- Touching the tip of the tongue to the palate just behind the front teeth

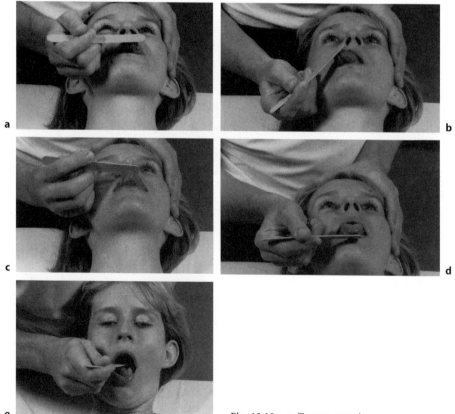

a

b

c

d

e   Fig. 13.18 a–e. Tongue exercises

13.4 Swallowing

Swallowing is a complex activity, controlled partly by voluntary action and partly by reflex activity (Kendall and McCreary 1983). Exercise can improve the action of the muscles involved in the reflex portion as well as in the voluntary portion of swallowing. Sitting, the functional eating position, is a practical position for exercising the muscles involved. Another good treatment position is prone on elbows.

Chewing is necessary to mix the food with saliva and shape it for swallowing. The tongue moves the food around within the mouth and then pushes the chewed food back to the pharynx with humping motions. To keep the food inside the mouth, patients must be able to hold their lips closed. Exercise of these facial and tongue motions is covered Sects. 13.2 and 13.3.

A hyperactive gag reflex will hinder swallowing. To help moderate this conditioned reflex, use prolonged gentle pressure on the tongue, preferably with a cold object. Start the pressure at the front of the tongue and work back toward the root. Simultaneous controlled breathing exercises will make the treatment more effective.

When the food reaches the back of the mouth and contacts the wall of the pharynx it triggers the reflex that controls the next part of the swallowing action. At the start of this phase the soft palate must elevate to close off the nasal portion of the pharynx. Facilitate this motion by stimulating the soft palate or uvula with a dampened swab. You can do this on both sides, or concentrate just on the weaker side.

As the swallowing activity continues, the hyoid bone and the larynx move upward. To stimulate the muscles that elevate the larynx use quick ice, ice sticks and stretch reflex. Give the stretch reflex diagonally down to the right and then to the left. Treat hyperactivity in these muscles with prolonged icing, relaxation techniques, and controlled breathing.

13.5 Speech Disorders

For satisfactory speech a person needs both proper motion of the face, mouth, and tongue and the ability to vary tone and control breathing. Patients who have only high vocal tones are helped by breathing exercises and ice over the laryngeal area. Patients with only low vocal tone benefit from stimulation of the laryngeal muscles with quick ice followed by stretch and resistance to the motion of laryngeal elevation.

Note: To prevent compression of the larynx or trachea apply pressure on only one side of the throat at a time (Fig. 13.19).

Promote controlled exhalation during speech with resisted breathing exercises (Sect. 13.6). Use Combination of Isotonics, starting with resisted inhalation (concentric contraction), followed by prolonged exhalation (resisted eccentric contraction of the muscles that enlarge the chest). During exhalation the patient recites words or counts as high as possible. Work on the patient's control of speech volume in the same way.

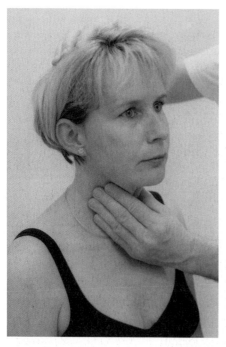

Fig. 13.19. Stimulation or relaxation of the throat

13.6 Breathing

Direct indications are breathing problems itself. Breathing problems can involve both breathing in (inhalation) and breathing out (exhalation). Treat the sternal, costal, and diaphragmatic areas to improve inspiration. Exercise the abdominal muscles to strengthen forced exhalation.

Indirect indications are for chest mobilization, trunk and shoulder mobility, active recuperation after exercise, relief of pain, relaxation and to decrease spasticity.

All the procedures and techniques are used in this area of care. Hand alignment is particularly important to guide the force in line with normal chest motion. Use the *stretch reflex* to facilitate the initiation of inhalation. Continue with Repeated Stretch through range (Repeated Contractions) to facilitate an increase in inspiratory volume. Appropriate resistance strengthens the muscles and guides the chest motion. Preventing motion on the stronger or more mobile side (timing for emphasis) will facilitate activity on the restricted or weaker side. Combination of Isotonics is useful when working on breath control. The patient should do breathing exercises in all positions. Emphasize treatment in functional positions.

Supine (Fig. 13.20)

- Place both hands on the sternum and apply oblique downward pressure (caudal and dorsal, towards the sacrum) (Fig. 13.20 a).
- Apply pressure on the lower ribs, diagonally in a caudal and medial direction, with both hands. Place your hands obliquely with the fingers following the line of the ribs (Fig. 13.20 b). Exercise the upper ribs in the same way, placing your hands on the pectoralis major muscles.

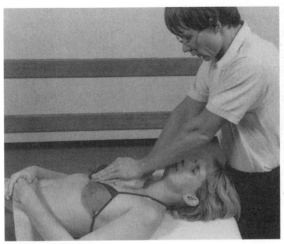
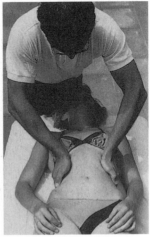

Fig. 13.20 a, b. Breathing in the supine position: **a** pressure on the sternum; **b** pressure on the lower ribs

Side Lying (Fig. 13.21)

- Use one hand on the sternum, the other on the back to stabilize and give counter pressure.
- Ribs: Put your hands on the area of the chest you wish to emphasize. Give the pressure diagonally in a caudal and medial direction to follow the line of the ribs. Point your fingers point in the same direction. In side lying the supporting surface will resist the motion of the other side of the chest).

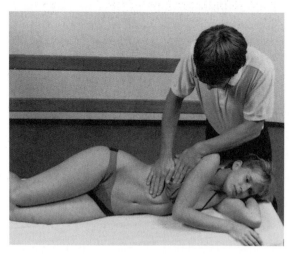

Fig. 13.21. Breathing in a side lying position

Prone (Fig. 13.22)

- Give pressure caudally along the line of the ribs. Place your hands on each side of the rib cage over the area to be emphasized. Your fingers follow the line of the ribs.

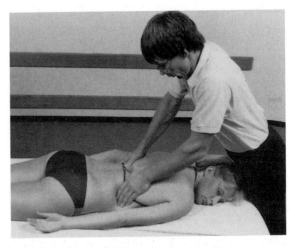

Fig. 13.22. Breathing in the prone position

Prone on Elbows (Fig. 13.23)

- Place one hand on the sternum and give pressure in a dorsal and caudal direction. Put your other hand on the spine at the same level for stabilizing pressure.
- Use the prone position hand placement and pressures.

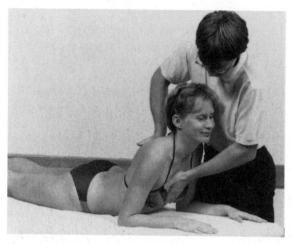

Fig. 13.23. Breathing in a prone position supported on the forearms

Facilitation of the Diaphragm (Fig. 13.24)

You can facilitate the diaphragm directly by pushing upward and laterally with the thumbs or fingers from below the rib cage (Fig. 13.24 a, b). Apply stretch and resist the downward motion of the contracting diaphragm. The patient's abdominal muscles must be relaxed for you to reach the diaphragm. If this is difficult, flex both hips to get more relaxation in the abdominal muscles and the hip flexor muscles. To give indirect facilitation for diaphragmatic motion, place your hands over the abdomen and ask the patient to inhale while pushing up into the gentle pressure (Fig. 13.24 c). Teach your patients to do this facilitation on their own.

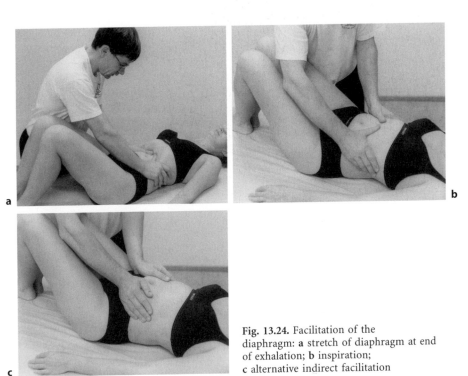

Fig. 13.24. Facilitation of the diaphragm: **a** stretch of diaphragm at end of exhalation; **b** inspiration; **c** alternative indirect facilitation

Reference

Kendall FP, McCreary EK (1983) Muscles, testing and function. Williams and Wilkins, Baltimore

14 Activities of Daily Living

Mastering the activities of daily living (ADL) is an important step in the patient's progress toward independence. The previous chapters have described a range of activities for achieving this goal: mat activities (rolling, bridging, crawling, kneeling, sitting), standing, walking, head and neck exercises, facial exercises, breathing, and swallowing.

When the patient has mastered the fundamentals needed for success in ADL, time may be spent working on more advanced or difficult activities. All the skills that a patient needs for independence can be taught using the PNF treatment approach. Guidance given by grip and resistance helps the patient develop effective ways to perform these activities.

Some of the practical activities are:
- Transferring from the wheelchair to bed (Fig. 14.1) and from bed to wheelchair (Fig. 14.2 d), onto the toilet (Fig. 14.2 a), into a shower, a bathtub (Fig. 14.2 b, c) a chair, a car, etc.
- Dressing and undressing (Fig. 14.3), washing.

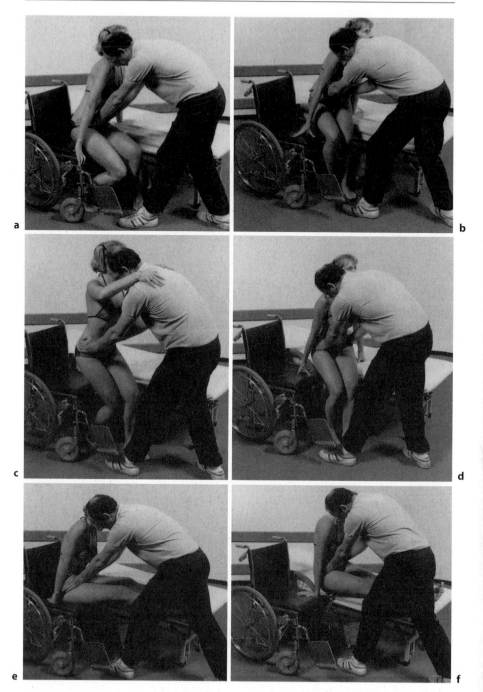

Fig. 14.1 a–f. Transfers from wheelchair to bed: guidance and resistance at pelvis

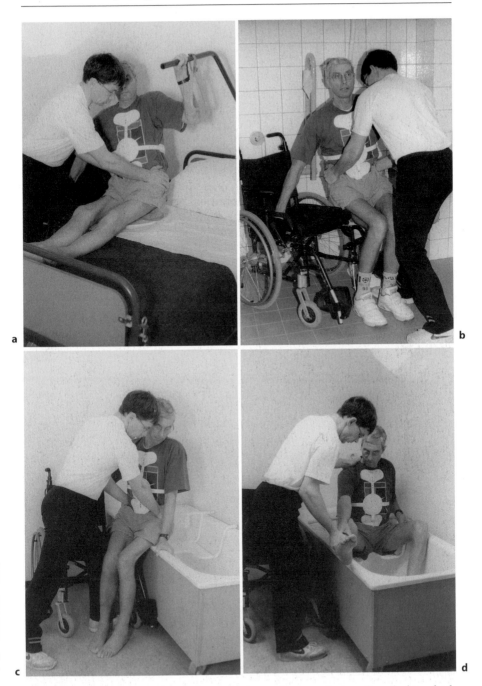

Fig. 14.2 a–d. Different transfers: patients with incomplete paraplegia. **a** From bed to wheelchair; **b** from wheelchair into toilet; **c, d** from wheelchair into bathtub

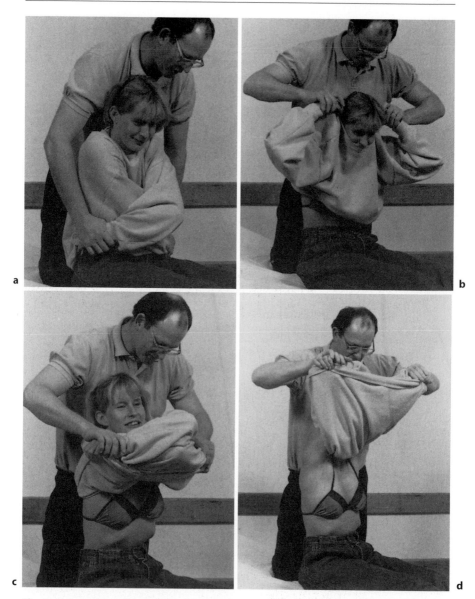

Fig. 14.3. Dressing and undressing. **a–d** taking shirt off, resistance to arms

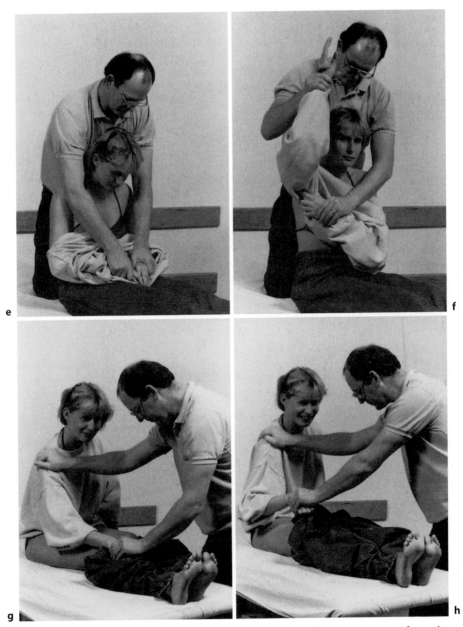

Fig. 14.3. Dressing and undressing. **e,f** putting shirt on, resistance to arms; **g,h** putting pants on, resistance to arms

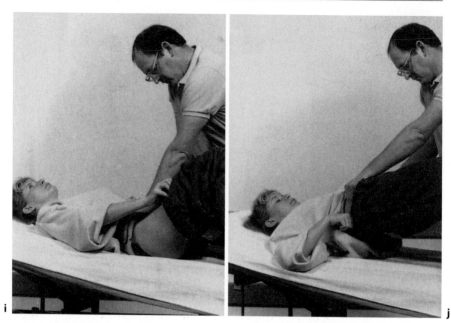

i   j

Fig. 14.3. Dressing and undressing. **i,j** putting pants on, resistance to bridging

15 Glossary

Afterdischarge

The effect of a stimulus, such as a muscle contraction, continues after the stimulus has stopped. The greater the stimulus the longer the afterdischarge.

Approximation

The compression of a segment or extremity through the long axis. The effect is to stimulate a muscular response and improve stability and postural muscle tonus.

Basic procedures (or principles)

A combination of different tools to facilitate and to increase the effectiveness of treatment.

Bilateral

On both body sides. Of both arms or both legs.

Bilateral asymmetrical

Moving both arms or both legs in opposite diagonals but in the same direction.
   Example: Right extremity, flexion–abduction; left extremity, flexion–adduction.

Bilateral symmetrical

Moving both arms or legs in the same diagonals and the same direction.
   Example: Right extremity, flexion–abduction; left extremity, flexion–abduction.

Bilateral symmetrical reciprocal

Moving both arms or legs in the same diagonals but in opposite directions.

Example: Right extremity, flexion–abduction; left extremity, extension–adduction.

Bilateral asymmetrical reciprocal

Moving both arms or legs in opposite diagonals and in opposite directions.

Example: Right extremity, flexion–adduction; left extremity, extension–adduction.

Chopping

Bilateral asymmetrical upper extremity extension with neck flexion to the same side to exercise the trunk flexor muscles (see Sect. 10.2.1)

Elongated state

The position in a pattern where all the muscles are under tension of elongation. Usually the starting position for the pattern.

Excitation

Activation or stimulation of muscular contractions. Promoting or encouraging motor activities.

Groove/diagonal

The line of movement in which a pattern takes place. Resistance is applied in this line of movement. The therapist's arms and body line up in this groove or diagonal. In most cases this line runs from one shoulder to the contralateral hip or is parallel to this line.

Hold

An isometric muscle contraction. No motion is attempted by the patient or the therapist.

Inhibition

Suppressing muscle contractions or nerve impulses.

Irradiation

The spread or increased force of a response that occurs when a stimulus is increased in strength or frequency. This ability is inherent to the neuromuscular system.

Lifting

Bilateral asymmetrical upper extremity flexion with neck extension to the same side to exercise trunk extension (see Sect. 10.2.2).

Lumbrical grip

A grip in which the lumbrical muscles are the prime movers. The metacarpal-phalangeal (MCP) joints flex and the proximal (PIP) and distal (DIP) interphalangeal joints remain relatively extended. Traction and rotational resistance are effectively applied with this hold.

Muscle contractions:

▶ Isotonic (dynamic): The intent of the patient is to produce motion.
  • Concentric: shortening of the agonist produces motion.
  • Eccentric: an outside force, gravity or resistance, produces the motion. The motion is restrained by the controlled lengthening of the agonist.
  • Stabilizing isotonic: the intent of the patient is motion, the motion is prevented by an outside force (usually resistance).
▶ Isometric (static): the intent of both the patient and the therapist is for no motion to occur.

Overflow

The expansion of a response. In therapy we make use of overflow from the stronger to the weaker parts of a pattern or from stronger patterns to weaker patterns of motion.

Pivot of action

The joint or body section in which movement takes place.

Reinforcement

The strengthening of a weaker segment by a stronger segment, which has been specially chosen for this purpose. It can work within a pattern or the reinforcement can come from another part of the body.

Repeated contractions

Eliciting the stretch reflex repeatedly from an already contracting muscle or muscles to produce stronger contractions.

Replication

A PNF technique to learn a movement or position.

Reversal

An agonistic motion followed by an antagonistic motion. This is an effective form of facilitation based on reciprocal innervation and successive induction.

Reciprocal Innervation

Excitation of the agonist is coupled with simultaneous inhibition of the antagonist. This provides a basis for coordinate movement.

Stretch

Elongation of muscular tissue.
▶ Stretch stimulus: increased excitation in muscles in the elongated state.
▶ Quick stretch: sharp stretch or tap on muscles under tension. A quick stretch is required to get a stretch reflex.
▶ Restretch: another quick stretch to a muscle that is under the tension of contraction.

Successive induction

Contraction of the antagonists is followed by an intensified excitation of the agonist. This is a basis for the reversal techniques.

Summation

The joining of subliminal stimuli resulting in excitation or a stronger contraction.
▶ Spatial summation: simultaneous stimuli from different parts of the body join to produce a stronger muscle contraction.
▶ Temporal summation: the combining of stimuli that occur within a short time period to produce a stronger muscle contraction or activate more motor units.

Technique

Resisted muscle contractions combined with appropriate facilitatory procedures to achieve specific objectives. The techniques are combined to achieve the desired results.

Timing

The sequencing of movements.
▶ Normal timing: the course or sequence of movements that results in coordinate movement.
▶ Timing for emphasis: changing the normal timing of movements to emphasize some component within the movement. This is especially effective when applying optimal resistance to stronger components within the movement.

Unilateral

On one side of the body. Of only one leg or arm.

Printing: Mercedes-Druck, Berlin
Binding: Stein+Lehmann, Berlin